Endovenous Laser Treatment of Varicose Veins: Practical Technique

Authors:

Dr. Manav Bhalla

and

Dr. Namrata Bhalla

Contributing Author:

Deepali Bhalla

Copyright © 2018 Manav Bhalla
All rights reserved.
ISBN-13: 9781719843966

PREFACE

Varicose veins are a global health problem that have a huge socio-economic impact, not restricted to territorial boundaries of any country of our world. Developed countries have a huge expenditure for annual as well long term care of this condition. This abnormal leg condition has various types of presentation and sometimes vague symptomatology. Identifying these symptoms and arriving at confirmed diagnosis is the first step to relieve this worldwide disease.

Traditionally, varicose veins have been managed surgically, which provided temporary symptomatic relief. This approach however has a high rate of recurrence and residual disease. With the introduction of newer interventional techniques, scenario of varicose veins management has entirely changed in past few years. The endovenous procedures, as they are commonly labeled, have not only improved the morbidity related to this disease, but also achieved a higher technical success rate.

Widely prevalent amongst such techniques has been the Endovenous Laser treatment. This procedure is performed across the globe in a variety of fashion, which basically comes down to same underlying mechanism of action. In skilled hands, though, the results may vary. However, anyone intending to perform this procedure may initially have innumerable questions pertaining to this disease and treatment techniques, some of which could be trivial and others critical.

We have been performing this procedure since 2005, and have been improvising our work with experience. Patients are our prime source of inspiration, and have made us more creative while dealing with their complex varicosities.

Taking a step forward, we also presented our work experience at national and international platform, namely Society of Interventional Radiology (SIR) in USA, European Congress of Radiology (ESR) in Austria, and Indian Radiological and Imaging Association (IRIA). In pursuit of acquiring new technical skills pertaining to our field, we signed up for advanced training programs in reputed institutions of United States. During these years, we had opportunity to interact with various physicians performing these procedures, and we found consistencies in technical results, although the procedures were performed in slightly different fashion, combination and timing.

With the aim that this procedure is understood easily and hopefully thoroughly by the beginners, health care practitioners, physicians, referring consultants, undergraduate and postgraduate medical students of various specialties and subspecialties, we have taken this step to write our experience. World over Interventional Radiologists perform this procedure, but scope of this procedure in India and some other countries, extends beyond the confines of Interventional Radiologists, to include subspecialties like general surgeons, vascular surgeons, cardiovascular surgeons, dermatologists, etc. For patients, we expect this book to provide insight into the normal anatomy and physiology of lower extremity venous system, a basic understanding of pathophysiology of chronic venous insufficiency, and hopefully and an overview of treatment approach.

One critical component of this as well as other endovenous procedures is ultrasound guidance, and hence the knowledge of vascular ultrasound, particularly venous exam is an unspoken requirement. If a physician performing this procedure is not verse with vascular ultrasound technique, utilizing services of a colleague radiologist or where appropriate, ultrasound technician is recommended.

We have tried to include the relevant information that one may found useful during the learning curve phase of the procedure, and serve as a valuable tool to refer to anytime later during practice. The book begins with abbreviations which are frequently used in this book, and are accepted by international communities. This is followed by lower limb venous anatomy, pathophysiology, clinical presentation and diagnoses of varicose veins. The detailed step in management of this condition by endovenous laser and sclerotherapy has then been explained, which includes the post procedure expectations.

It is our sincere wish that this book motivates readers by filling in the technical information gap that prevents successful outcomes. Any questions are most welcome. We will try to answer those to the best of our abilities.

Sincerely,

Namrata Bhalla   Manav Bhalla

ACKNOWLEDGEMENT

Treating our patients has been the source of inspiration for us. They have immensely contributed towards our learning experience.

Sincere thanks to our daughter, Deepali Bhalla, who has contributed immensely to this book. In our clinical practice, we utilized sketches, diagrams and models made by her, to explain the patients. We have incorporated some of those sketches here in this book.

The sketch below and at the end of book is from Deepali. Both the sketches are same, the initial one is inverse of the latter. Initial inverse sketch represents how venous network is organized to allow central directional flow from tributaries to main veins, that goes haywire in varicose veins. It's our skillful task to streamline the flow as best we can. The subsequent sketch is of a beautiful tree.

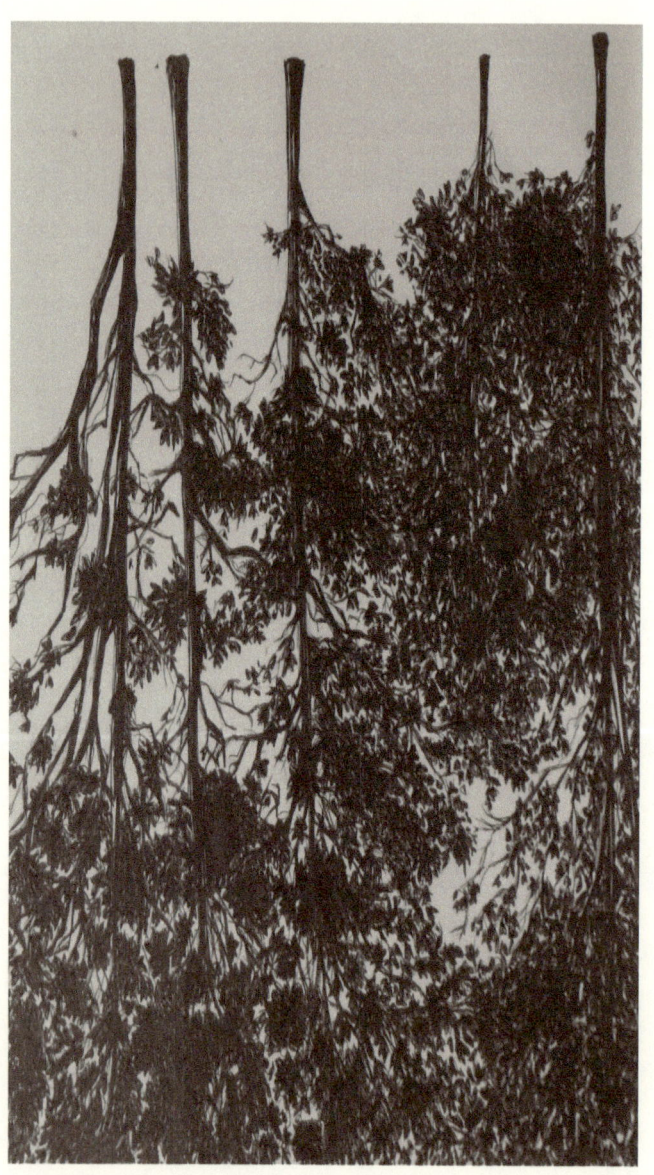

ABBREVIATIONS OR TERMINOLOGIES USED IN THIS BOOK

AASV: Anterior accessory saphenous vein
ATV: Anterior tibial vein
AVP: Ambulatory venous pressure
CD: Color Doppler
CEAP: clinical manifestations (C), etiologic factors (E), anatomic distribution of disease (A), and underlying pathophysiologic findings (P).
CVI: Chronic Venous insufficiency
DVT: Deep venous thrombosis.
EVL: Endovenous Laser.
EFIT: Endovenous foam-induced thrombus.
EHIT: Endothermal heat-induced thrombosis.
GSV: Greater Saphenous Vein (or previously known as Long saphenous vein)
IVC: Inferior Vena Cava
PASV: Posterior accessory saphenous vein
PTV: Posterior tibial vein
PW: Pulse wave (Doppler)
RFA: Radiofrequency Ablation.
SFJ: Sapheno-femoral junction
SN: Saphenous nerve
SPJ: Sapheno-popliteal junction
SSV: Short saphenous vein (or previously known as lesser saphenous vein)
Ulcus cruris: Venous ulcers, venous insufficiency ulceration, stasis ulcers, stasis dermatitis, varicose ulcers
US: Ultrasound
VCSS: Venous clinical severity score

Table of Contents

PREFACE 2
ACKNOWLEDGEMENT 5
ABBREVIATIONS OR TERMINOLOGIES USED IN THIS BOOK 7
1. LOWER LIMB VENOUS ANATOMY 9
2. PATHOPHYSIOLOGY OF VARICOSE VEINS 26
3. CLINICAL PRESENTATION 41
4. ULTRASOUND IMAGING 55
5. MANAGEMENT TECHNIQUES 74
6. PATIENT SELECTION FOR ENDOVENOUS LASER 88
7. CONCEPT OF LASER APPLICATION IN VARICOSE VEINS TREATMENT 92
8. PRE-OPERATIVE WORK UP PRIOR TO ENDOVENOUS LASER 100
9. ENDOVENOUS LASER TECHNIQUE 106
10. SCLEROTHERAPY 131
11. POST PROCEDURE MANAGEMENT AND FOLLOW UP 146
12. EXPECTED OUTCOMES, RESULTS, AND POSSIBLE COMPLIATIONS 153
13. RECURRENCE OF VARICOSE VEINS 162
Conclusion 166

Chapter 1

LOWER LIMB VENOUS ANATOMY

INTRODUCTION

The nomenclature adopted in this book is as per the International interdisciplinary consensus statement on nomenclature of lower limbs veins.[1]

This chapter is intended to provide a brief overview of lower limb venous anatomy which in our experience is relevant to the endovenous procedure. For the detailed anatomical knowledge, readers are recommended to refer to a dedicated literature.

Lower limb venous system includes the deep venous system, superficial venous system, and perforators (see table 1.1). As the name implies, deep system includes veins situated deeper to the muscular fascia, and superficial system includes veins located superficial to muscular fascia.[17] A third and vital component of lower extremity venous system is the perforating venous system, which interconnects the deep and superficial venous system by traversing the muscular fascia which divides these two systems. Additionally, there are communicating veins which interconnect the veins across the same plane or system, i.e., communicating a superficial vein to another superficial vein in the same plane, or communicating a deep vein to another deep vein in the same plane.

Initial presentation of diseases involving these venous systems (superficial versus deep) have different clinical presentations, although later during the progressive course of untreated disease, both the systems may be involved, resulting in considerable overlap of signs and symptoms.

CHARACTERISTICS OF LOWER EXTREMITY VEINS

The venous wall has 3 layers: intima, media, and adventitia.[18,19] Numerous bicuspid valves are present in the lower extremity veins, which are folds of endothelium, supported by connective tissue.[20] Primary function of the valves is to aid in antegrade flow of venous return towards the heart.[21] Numbers of valves within the veins are variable, being relatively more distally (or peripherally) compared to proximal (or central) locations, being less as we move towards groin. Valves and surrounding calf musculature aid in antegrade blood flow, which essentially means flow from superficial to deep venous system and from peripheral to central aspect of venous system.

UNDERSTANDING VENOUS CIRCUIT

Table 1.1. Constituents of Lower limb venous system

Superficial (*superficial to muscular fascia*)	Deep (*deep to muscular fascia*)
• Greater Saphenous vein (GSV) • Short saphenous vein (SSV) • Reticular veins	• Common femoral vein (CFV) • Femoral vein (FV) • Profunda • Popliteal • Anterior tibial veins (ATV), paired • Posterior tibial veins (PTV), paired • Peroneal veins, paired • Gastrocnemius • Soleal
Perforator (*interconnects superficial and deep system, traverses muscular fascia*) Direct Indirect	

Communicating (*connecting veins situated within same planes, do not traverse muscular fascia*)

The traditional labeling of a vein's location in the lower extremity, as "proximal" and "distal" can be confusing. For example, a segment of vein within the distal leg could be a distal vein. However, in terms of flow direction, that particular segment of vein could be proximal in the venous circuit, since it receives venous blood prior to a segment of vein located in groin. For that matter, if the flowing stream of water represents venous blood flow, the segment of vein in distal leg could be considered as upstream location and the segment of vein in groin may be considered as downstream location, albeit in relative terms. As the venous blood advances further, this segment of vein in groin becomes upstream in location when compared to segment of vein in abdomen (IVC).

Now, to keep things consistent in understanding, we can adopt a uniform way of naming these vein locations. The venous circuit located upstream, i.e. far away from right atrium (which is the epicenter for receiving venous return) is called peripheral. And the segment of vein closer to right atrium can be called central. To illustrate, let's take an example of a stream of water representing femoral vein in thigh (see Sketch 1.2). The femoral vein in distal thigh could be labeled as peripheral portion of femoral vein, and the segment of femoral vein located in proximal thigh, could be labeled as central portion of femoral vein. Even though these terms, central and peripheral, are relative, they reflect the directional venous circuit.

Now, let's look at the individual systems which constitute the lower extremity venous circuit.

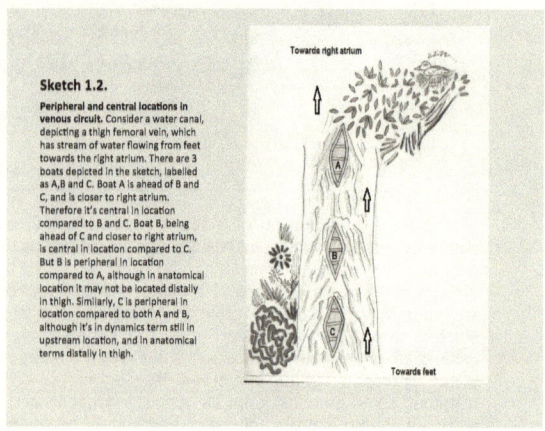

Sketch 1.2.

Peripheral and central locations in venous circuit. Consider a water canal, depicting a thigh femoral vein, which has stream of water flowing from feet towards the right atrium. There are 3 boats depicted in the sketch, labelled as A,B and C. Boat A is ahead of B and C, and is closer to right atrium. Therefore it's central in location compared to B and C. Boat B, being ahead of C and closer to right atrium, is central in location compared to C. But B is peripheral in location compared to A, although in anatomical location it may not be located distally in thigh. Similarly, C is peripheral in location compared to both A and B, although it's in dynamics term still in upstream location, and in anatomical terms distally in thigh.

DEEP VENOUS SYSTEM

Components of deep venous system

The deep venous system involves common femoral vein (CFV), femoral vein (FV), profunda, popliteal vein, and calf veins. The calf veins include soleal, gastrocnemius, peroneal, anterior tibial (ATV) and posterior tibial veins (PTV) (see Sketch 1.3).

The gastrocnemius veins drain the medial and lateral gastrocnemius muscles, and ultimately drains into the popliteal vein.[4] The soleal veins drain into SSV or popliteal vein. The gastrocnemius and soleal veins play an important role in the calf muscle pump function. The paired anterior tibial, posterior tibial, and peroneal veins are the venae comitantes of the corresponding arteries, and drain into popliteal vein.

The term "superficial femoral vein" has been replaced by "femoral vein", per current nomenculature.[1] The femoral and profunda femoral veins join to form common femoral vein. The CFV drains into external iliac vein.

Direction of flow in deep venous system

The normal physiological direction of blood flow is peripheral (i.e. foot) to central (towards groin and ultimately towards right atrium). In an erect standing patient, this is anti-gravitational direction.

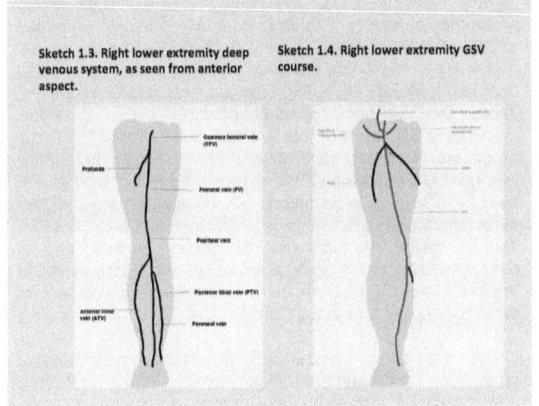

Sketch 1.3. Right lower extremity deep venous system, as seen from anterior aspect.

Sketch 1.4. Right lower extremity GSV course.

SUPERFICIAL VENOUS SYSTEM

Components of superficial venous system

The components are Greater Saphenous vein (GSV), Short saphenous vein (SSV) and reticular veins. As per the international consensus, the terms long or internal saphenous vein have been replaced by Great saphenous vein (GSV), and the terms lesser or short saphenous vein or external saphenous vein have been replaced by Small saphenous vein (SSV).

Greater Saphenous Vein (GSV) – course and tributaries

Greater Saphenous vein begins its course from the medial aspect of dorsal venous arch of foot, courses anterior to medial malleolus, localizing in anteromedial aspect of leg, thereafter coursing (see sketch 1.4) postero-medially somewhere in proximal one third of leg. It courses medially at the level of knee and then can be traced along anteromedial aspect of thigh to be finally localized at medial aspect of anterior groin where it is seen piercing the fascia, and finally draining into the deep venous system, namely the common femoral vein (CFV). The junction of GSV and CFV, called the Sapheno femoral junction (SFJ) is worth mentioning for some important reasons pertaining to this procedure. The SFJ has valve which promotes antegrade flow from GSV into the CFV and prevent reflux of flow at rest as well as strenuous conditions like Valsalva's maneuver. An initial short period of reflux is physiological which is < 0.5 second, better demonstrated on duplex studies, and is described later in the book. Also, as we will discuss later in the book, this SFJ serves as a landmark for placement of laser fiber tip within the GSV lumen.

The saphenous compartment is a sub compartment of superficial compartment (see sketch 1.5), bordered superficially by saphenous fascia (appearing hyperechoic on ultrasound) and deeply by the muscular fascia. [3,4] The great saphenous vein usually lies directly on the muscular fascia in the saphenous compartment. The saphenous compartment contains the saphenous vein and the accompanying arteries and nerves. Important landmark to remember is that the only truncal vein located within saphenous compartment is GSV or its duplicate (see caption 1.6). The tributaries of GSV, any accessory, collateral or communicating veins lie external to this compartment [1,2,3]. The saphenous compartment has "Egyptian eye" appearance on ultrasound.

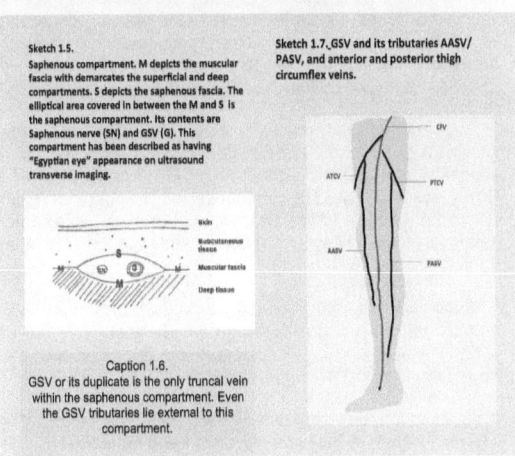

Sketch 1.5.
Saphenous compartment. M depicts the muscular fascia with demarcates the superficial and deep compartments. S depicts the saphenous fascia. The elliptical area covered in between the M and S is the saphenous compartment. Its contents are Saphenous nerve (SN) and GSV (G). This compartment has been described as having "Egyptian eye" appearance on ultrasound transverse imaging.

Sketch 1.7. GSV and its tributaries AASV/ PASV, and anterior and posterior thigh circumflex veins.

Caption 1.6.
GSV or its duplicate is the only truncal vein within the saphenous compartment. Even the GSV tributaries lie external to this compartment.

Tributaries of GSV:
It is important to note that besides the tributaries mentioned below, there may be variations in normal anatomy. Additionally, in chronic venous insufficiency there may be presence of varying number of venous channels which are identified on venous mapping by ultrasound. Since these may be important in the pathophysiology of chronic

venous disease, they may also need attention during treatment.

Accessory great saphenous vein indicates vein ascending parallel to GSV in leg and thigh (see sketch 1.7). The anterior accessory saphenous vein (AASV) refers to a venous segment located anteriorly within a fascial compartment in the thigh.[6] The posterior accessory saphenous vein (PASV) refers to a venous segment located posteriorly within a fascial compartment in the thigh. This vein is not found as often as the AASV and its connection with GSV is not constant.[6] The leg segment of posterior accessory saphenous vein corresponds to the so-called *Leonardo's vein* or *Posterior arch vein*.

The anterior and posterior thigh circumflex veins are localized in anterior and posterior thigh as the name suggests, and may be tributaries for GSV itself or AASV / PASV respectively. The tributaries of the anterior thigh circumflex vein are located laterally in the thigh, which unite and enlarge as they course obliquely and then form the main trunk to join its draining vein.

Superficial external pudendal, superficial circumflex iliac, and superficial epigastric veins that drain the lower abdominal wall and perineum drain into the GSV near the SFJ.[2] (see sketch 1.4).

Intersaphenous veins: One or more intersaphenous veins course obliquely in the leg to connect the SSV and GSV.

The lateral venous system localized in lateral aspect of thigh and leg also drains into GSV. Abnormal development of this system may be found in patients with Klippel-Trenaunay syndrome.[4]

True GSV duplication consists of identifying splitting of the vein into two channels, both lying on the muscular fascia, which later rejoin. It is seen in the thigh in 8%[3] and in the calf in 25% of the cases.

Facts to remember (see caption 1.8)
Saphenous nerve is usually far from the great saphenous vein (GSV), however it lies in close proximity to the GSV distal to the Knee.[4] This relation is clinically very important to remember while delivering the laser energy to this segment of the superficial vein, since the adjoining nerve may be at risk of injury and could potentially cause tingling, numbness or pain in treated leg. Besides thermal damage, other possible causes that can injure the saphenous nerve (or for that matter Sural nerve which is seen in relation with Short saphenous vein) are: needle injury during vein access or while administering the tumescent local anesthesia.

A terminal valve is usually localized in GSV 1-2 mm peripheral to the SFJ in 94%–100% of the cases.[7] Another preterminal valve is seen 2 cm peripheral to the previously mentioned valve. Needless to say, there can be variations in the locations of these valves, and these could be congenitally absent.[22,23] Anatomic and ultrasound relevance of these valves is that some important tributaries drain into intervening segment of GSV between these two valves.

The medial and lateral plantar veins, deep plantar venous arch, deep metatarsal and deep digital veins (plantar and dorsal), and pedal veins are considered deep veins. The anatomic origin of GSV and SSV, namely the dorsal venous arch, and medial and lateral marginal veins are considered superficial.[1] Varicose veins in the medial and lateral retro malleolar space are also subcutaneous tributaries of the GSV and SSV, respectively.[6]

Chart 1.8. Facts to remember

GSV
- Saphenous nerve courses closer to GSV, below knee.
- Terminal and preterminal GSV valves
- Plantar veins are considered deep veins, except for the origins of GSV and SSV, which are considered superficial.
- Retromalleolar veins are classified superficial.

SSV
Sural nerve proximity to SSV, the latter being medially situated.

Perforator
The foot perforators are an exception as they normally have bidirectional flow.

Small saphenous vein (SSV) – course and tributaries

The SSV arises from lateral aspect of dorsal pedal arch, ascend posterior to the lateral malleolus, coursing posteriorly in superficial compartment of calf, and then terminating variably in popliteal vein. The termination of SSV into popliteal vein is termed sapheno-popliteal junction (SPJ), which most often lies 2–4 cm above the popliteal skin crease but its exact location is variable.[6,10] The drainage of SSV may be seen into the GSV via anterior or posterior tributaries, or into the femoral, deep femoral or internal iliac veins. (see sketch 1.9).

The SSV may extend cranially in posterior thigh, localizing itself in the groove between the biceps femoris and semimembranosus muscles. It has been called the 'femoropopliteal vein' or cranial extension of the SSV and it terminates in one or more superficial or perforating veins of the thigh or gluteal region.[9] However, the cranial extension of SSV may communicate with GSV through posterior thigh circumflex vein, often then referred to as vein of Giacomini.[1]

The SSV may also communicate with the medial ankle perforators through several tributaries.[3] Other alternative drainage pathways through the internal iliac system, inferior gluteal veins, obturator veins, and along the round ligament have been described.[2]

Tributaries of SSV:
The lateral arch vein is the major tributary of the small saphenous vein.
Facts to remember
The SSV lies medial to and in close proximity to the sural nerve. (see sketch 1.10)

Reticular veins
They are extensive network of veins situated beneath the skin, within the superficial compartment but superficial to the saphenous fascia. These veins are responsible for draining the skin and subcutaneous tissue of lower extremity.[2] These reticular veins may drain into saphenous tributaries or deep veins through perforators, the latter have been reported in patients with extensive telangiectasia.[2]

Sketch 1.9 : Short Saphenous vein course in posterior calf

Sketch 1.10. Sural nerve. Medial sural cutaneous nerve (MSCN) which is branch of tibial nerve is the major contributor for sural nerve. Peroneal communicating, a branch of lateral sural cutaneous nerve (LSCN), which in turn is a branch of common peroneal nerve, usually communicates with MSCN to form Sural nerve. Please note, this is just a sketch of nerve course, and not a graphed distance from SSV.

PERFORATING VENOUS SYSTEM

Perforators, as the name imply, perforate the muscular fascia, and traverse both the superficial and deep compartments. Perforators that connect a superficial vein to the deep vein are called the **direct perforators**. The perforators, which join the superficial vein to the veins within the muscle, are **indirect perforators**.

The perforators contain valves and they demonstrate unidirectional blood flow, i.e. superficial to deep. Incompetence of these perforating vein valves may contribute to venous congestion, varicosities, and chronic skin changes including ulceration.[8] The foot perforators are an exception as they normally have bidirectional flow.

Groups of perforators

Perforators are grouped based on their topography.[1]

Foot perforators[11] : Medial, lateral, dorsal and plantar.

Ankle perforators[11] : Medial, lateral and anterior.

Calf perforators:
- Medial leg perforators – Paratibial perforators (connect main GSV trunk or its tributaries to posterior tibial vein or calf muscle plexus) and posterior tibial perforators (connect posterior arch vein with posterior tibial veins).
- Anterior leg perforators – connect anterior GSV tributaries to anterior tibial vein
- Lateral leg perforators – connect lateral venous plexus to peroneal veins.
- Posterior leg perforators – Medial gastrocnemius perforator, lateral gastrocnemius perforator, intergemellar (soleal) perforator (connects SSV with soleal

veins), and para-Achillean perforator (connects SSV with peroneal veins).

The medial calf perforators, namely the paratibial and posterior tibial perforators, are clinically most important. Eponyms associated with the paratibial (Boyd perforators in upper leg and Sherman perforators in upper and mid leg) and posterior tibial perforators (Cockett perforators) should no longer be used.[1] Most occur along a 3-cm-wide lane ascending the medial calf, surrounding what has been called "Linton's line."[7]

Knee perforators: medial, lateral, suprapatellar, infrapatellar, popliteal fossa

Thigh perforators:
- Medial thigh perforators– femoral canal (previously called Dodd perforator) and inguinal perforators; connect GSV or its tributaries with femoral vein.
- Anterior thigh perforator.
- Lateral thigh perforator.
- Posterior thigh perforator.
- Pudendal perforator.

Gluteal perforators: superior gluteal, mid gluteal and lower gluteal perforators.

SAPHENOUS NERVE AND ITS RELATION TO GSV

The saphenous nerve (SN) needs special mention in the chapter of venous anatomy, since its proximity to the GSV makes it vulnerable to damage not only during surgical procedures, but also the endovascular techniques.

Saphenous nerve is a purely sensory nerve, which originates from femoral nerve (L3,4), and is primarily responsible for supplying medial side of lower leg. It usually becomes subcutaneous at the level of knee, piercing the deep fascia between tendons of Sartorius and gracilis.[13]

Veverkova et al described the anatomical relations between saphenous nerve and the GSV.[12] In majority of the cases, SN and GSV shared thin connective tissue sheath, which surrounded them. The nerve and sheath were separated by thin connective tissue lamella, but in some of the cases it was absent and there was a gap (of < 0.8 cm) noted in between them. There is no statistical significant difference noted in the median distance between the SN and GSV in proximal/distal versus mid leg, but they were relatively shorter in proximal and distal leg segments i.e., in the histological assessment of their set of patients they found SN to be closer to GSV in proximal and distal leg, as compared to the mid leg.[12]

The nerve in majority of patients lie posterior to the GSV, especially in the proximal and middle third leg, but is localized anterior to the vein in distal third of leg.

Damage to SN can cause sensation loss, permanent or temporary, and has been discussed in later chapters. Interestingly, nerve avulsion was noted in surgical stripping of GSV carried out in upwards stripping manner, and not in downward stripping.[13]

SURAL NERVE AND ITS RELATION TO SSV[14]

The Sural nerve is closely related to SSV, and so needs to be considered while managing the venous insufficiency associated with SSV.

There is great deal of variation in sural nerve components. Medial sural cutaneous nerve (MSCN) always forms sural nerve. It originates from the tibial nerve in popliteal fossa, descends between the heads of gastrocnemius muscles, deep to the fascia, and become superficial at junction of mid and distal third of leg.[16] The lateral sural cutaneous nerve (LSCN) originates from common peroneal nerve, and gives off peroneal communicating branch, which usually joins the MSCN where it penetrates the fascia, to form sural nerve. The MSCN by itself may form the sural nerve without contributions from LSCN, in approximately 20 % cases. [16] (See Sketch 1.10)

Sural nerve is located lateral to SSV, and courses 1-1.5 cm posterior to lateral malleolus.[16] Although there is significant variability in the distance between SSV and sural nerve, the distance is < 5mm in proximal one-third leg in 70% of the cases, and < 5 mm in distal two-third leg in 90% of the cases. There is fascia present between the vein and nerve in proximal one-third leg, that acts as a natural barrier, but is absent distally. Therefore, the proximal one-third is the optimal zone for ablation, in terms of avoiding nerve damage. This does not come without a caution, which is the extent of ablation that can be performed in this SSV. As we move centrally along the SSV, there are nerves (Tibial nerve and common peroneal nerve) which are closer to the SPJ, which then are at risk of thermal damage.

Sural nerve injury may lead to numbness, paresthesia, anesthesia along the nerve distribution, which typically is along posterolateral surface of leg and lateral border of foot. The evolution of nerve injury into neuroma may cause radiating pain to forefoot, and constant burning and painful paresthesia.[15] Ultrasound can be used effectively to identify sural nerve in posterior calf and thereby has potential to prevent damage.[15]

REFERENCES:

1. Caggiati A, Bergan JJ, Gloviczki P, Jantet G, Wendell-Smith CP, Partsch H. Nomenclature of the veins of the lower limbs: an international interdisciplinary consensus statement. J Vasc Surg 2002;36:416–422
2. Somjen GM. Anatomy of the superficial venous system.Dermatol Surg 1995;21:35–45

3. Thomson H. The surgical anatomy of the superficial and perforating veins of the lower limb. Ann R Coll Surg Engl 1979;61:198–205
4. Levent Oğuzkur. Ultrasonographic anatomy of the lower extremity superficial veins. Diagn Interv Radiol 2012; 18:423–430
5. Caggiati A. Fascial relations and structure of the tributaries of the saphenous veins. Surg Radiol Anat 2000;22:191-6.
6. Cavezzi A, Labropoulos N, Partsch H, et al. Duplex ultrasound investigation of the veins in chronic venous disease of the lower limbs-UIP consensus document. Part II. Anatomy. Eur J Vasc Endovasc Surg 2006; 31:288–299.
7. Meissner MH. Lower extremity venous anatomy. Semin Intervent Radiol 2005; 22:147–156.
8. Meissner, Mark H. et al. The hemodynamics and diagnosis of venous disease. J Vasc Surg 2007; 46(6): S4 - S24
9. Georgiev M. The femoropopliteal vein. Derm Surg 1996;22:57-62.
10. Myers KA, Wood SR, Lee V, Koh P. Variations of connections to the saphenous system in limbs with primary varicose veins: a study in 1481 limbs by duplex ultrasound scanning. J Phlebol 2002;2:11–17.
11. Kuster G, Lofgren EP, Hollinshead WH. Anatomy of the veins of the foot. Surg Gynecol Obstet 1968;127:817-26.
12. L Veverkova´, VJedlic˘ka, PVlc˘ek andJKalac.The anatomical relationship between the saphenous nerve and the great saphenous vein. Phlebology 2011;26:114–118
13. Ramasastry SS, Dick GO, Futrell JW. Anatomy of the saphenous nerve: relevance to saphenous vein stripping. Am Surg. 1987 May;53(5):274-7.
14. Kerver AL, van der Ham AC, Theeuwes HP, Eilers PH, Poublon AR, Kerver AJ, Kleinrensink GJ. The surgical anatomy of the small saphenous vein and adjacent nerves in relation to endovenous thermal ablation. J Vasc Surg. 2012 Jul;56(1):181-8.

15. Ricci S[1], Moro L, Antonelli Incalzi R. Ultrasound imaging of the sural nerve: ultrasound anatomy and rationale for investigation. Eur J Vasc Endovasc Surg. 2010 May;39(5):636-41
16. Ortigüela ME, Wood MB, Cahill DR. Anatomy of the sural nerve complex. J Hand Surg Am. 1987 Nov;12(6):1119-23.
17. Hollinshead WH. The back and limbs. In: Hollinshead WH, ed. Anatomy for surgeons. New York: Harper & Row Publishers. 1969. 617-631, 754-758, 803-807
18. Moneta G L, Nehler M R. In: Gloviczki P, Yao JST, editor. Handbook of Venous Disorders: Guidelines of the American Venous Forum. 1st ed. London: Chapman and Hall Medical; 1996. The lower extremity venous system: anatomy and physiology of normal venous function and chronic venous insufficiency. pp. 3–26.
19. Nichols JB, Vale FP. Histology and pathology: A manual for students and practitioners. Lea brothers&co. p.79.
20. Shapir O, Lev M. The venous valve in the aged. *Am Heart J.* 1952;44:843-850.
21. Hochauf S, Sternitzky R, Schellong SM. Struktur und Funktion des venösen Systems. Herz 2007;32:3-9 TERMINAL VALVES Dominic Mühlberger, Luca Morandini, Erich Brenner, Venous valves and major superficial tributary veins near the saphenofemoral junction, Journal of Vascular Surgery, Volume 49, Issue 6, June 2009, Pages 1562-1569.
22. Dominic Mühlberger, Luca Morandini, Erich Brenner, Venous valves and major superficial tributary veins near the saphenofemoral junction, Journal of Vascular Surgery, Volume 49, Issue 6, June 2009, Pages 1562-1569
23. Dominic Mühlberger, Luca Morandini, Erich Brenner, An anatomical study of femoral vein valves near the saphenofemoral junction, Journal of Vascular Surgery, Volume 48, Issue 4, October 2008, Pages 994-999

Chapter 2

PATHOPHYSIOLOGY OF VARICOSE VEINS

Chapter facts to remember (see chart 2.1 – 2.5)

The goal of embryological designed lower limb venous framework is to provide effective venous return from superficial to deep system, and caudal to cephalad-directed flow, thereby returning the venous blood towards right atrium. This goal is achieved by number of factors, which include:

1. **Presence of framework of veins** itself, i.e. absence of any one of them sets up a potential for ineffective venous return. The extreme example of this is seen in Klippel–Trénaunay syndrome, although manifestations may be theoretically more commonly seen in patients with stripped greater saphenous vein.
2. **Effective bicuspid venous valves.** The absence of valves or damage to these valves, the latter seen most commonly secondary to venous thrombosis, sets up the stage for venous insufficiency. The valves may be rendered incompetent by degenerative processes as well.
3. **Muscular venous pumps.** We will have a brief discussion of this later in the chapter.

The opposition to venous return in standing position though is provided by hydrostatic pressure of blood column, as well as the gravitational pull.

STRUCTURES RESPONSIBLE FOR ANTEGRADE VENOUS RETURN

Let's have a look at what mechanisms make venous return happen, which will then help us understand the events that happen in way of developing varicose veins.

VENOUS FRAMEWORK

To begin with, we require at least the skeletal presence of venous network in the lower limb, and it's centrally draining outlet/pathway. Obviously, deviation from the normal routes of venous flow could result in some alteration in flow dynamics.

Abnormalities which may be noted in this category are:

a. Absence of a vein.[2]
b. Surgical removal of vein.
c. Presence of GSV but not in the saphenous compartment.[1]

Chart 2.1. Facts to remember

Requirement for normal lower extremity venous return
- Presence of intact Venous framework
- Competent Venous valves
- Functionally efficient Musculovenous pumps.

Opponents of venous return.
- Gravity
- Hydrostatic pressure of blood column

Pathologic reflux : Retrograde flow > 0.5 seconds

Chart 2.2. Facts to remember

- Proximal compression on ultrasound does not differentiate normal from abnormal venous reflux.

- Valsalva's maneuver is good for evaluation of iliofemoral segments only.

- Distal veins are better evaluated using release of distal compression, in a standing patient.

Chart 2.3. Facts to remember

Primary venous insufficiency

- Cause unknown
- Venous wall dilatation leads to reflux (wall changes precede reflux)
- Affected veins : GSV, its tributaries and perforators
- Deep veins less commonly affected
- Multi-centric involvement
- Reflux is the only hemodynamic abnormality

Chart 2.4. Facts to remember

Secondary venous insufficiency

- Can be caused by :
  ✓ Post thrombotic valvular damage (leading to reflux)
  ✓ Venous obstruction

- Affected veins : Superficial, deep, perforators

- Progression potentiated by : Calf muscle pump dysfunction.

- Reflux and obstruction could both be the hemodynamic abnormality.

Klippel–Trénaunay syndrome is a rare congenital medical condition in which blood vessels and/or lymph vessels fail to form properly. The three main features are nevus flammeus (port-wine stain), venous and lymphatic malformations, and soft-tissue hypertrophy of the affected limb. It could be associated with aplasia of GSV^3, or left iliac vein aplasia[2].

Chart 2.5. Facts to remember

Chronic venous insufficiency

- Venous refill time decreases
- AVP increases
- Linear relation between ulcer incidence and AVP > 30 mmHg
- Ulcer incidence increases with venous filling > 7 mL/sec
- Clinical manifestation : leg edema, pigmentation, ulceration, fibrosis

Pittaluga et al[1] observed that the absence of GSV in the saphenous compartment at the mid-thigh was associated with a younger age and a higher body mass index, with a higher frequency of symptoms, edema, and skin changes in patients with chronic venous insufficiency.

VENOUS VALVES

There are numerous valves present within the venous system as mentioned in chapter on anatomy.

In a resting supine position, the valves remain open and the venous blood normally flows antegrade from a high-pressure venous segment to low-pressure venous segment (typically peripheral to central), due to the pressure gradient across the valve.

In the standing state or in a situation when the pressure gradient does not exist, i.e., the pressure across the valve equalizes, there is venous stasis, and there is neither the antegrade nor retrograde flow. The valves remain open.

With the subsequent reversal in pressure gradient, the pressure central to the valve is higher and peripheral to the valve is lower, resulting in reversal of flow i.e. retrograde flow. The valve remains open. Only when the retrograde flow achieves a certain velocity, do the valves close. This velocity is approximately 30 cm/sec. Once the valves close, they act as barriers and divide the hydrostatic column of blood into segments. (see sketch 2.6).

The take home point from this physiological phenomenon is [4]: The short period of reversal of flow prior to valve closure is therefore normal physiologic flow reversal, and approximately lasts for 0.5 seconds. The reflux is considered pathological if the retrograde flow persists for more than 0.5 seconds. However, Labropoulus et al, based on their study suggested that although cut off value for reflux in superficial

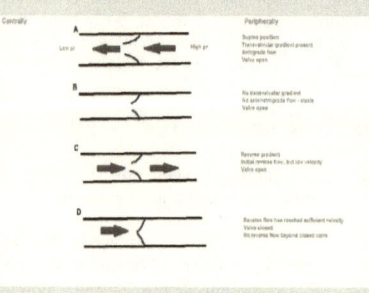

Sketch 2.6. Pressure gradients across venous valve and normal valve closure. Note that the events B-D can occur in situations like erect position or proximal external compression.

veins, deep femoral vein and deep calf vein is > 500 ms (or 0.5 sec), the cut off for reflux in femoropopliteal veins should be > 1000 ms (or 1 sec), and that in perforators it should be > 350 ms. Additionally, they suggested that reflux evaluation on ultrasound should be performed in standing position only, and not in supine position.

Cessation of antegrade flow does not cause or results from the valve closure. This is an important physiologic concept to understand.

Let's now take a look at the relevance of the clinical maneuver's we commonly perform on these patient's: External compression and Valsalva's maneuver.

Proximal external compression
In a supine patient, proximal compression causes retrograde pressure gradient which is not sufficient to cause velocity of 30 cm/sec. As a result, the valvular leaflets do not appose, and the reflux of venous blood persists. Therefore, evaluation of venous reflux on ultrasound using proximal compression in a supine patient will normally reveal a reflux, and not differentiate from abnormal reflux, rendering this this technique non-viable option for reflux evaluation a non-viable option.

Valsalva's maneuver
This maneuver produces reversal of pressure gradient across the valves, which is sufficient to cause reversal of blood velocity and the subsequent valve closure in the iliofemoral segments only, but not peripherally. So, the distal femoral, profunda, popliteal and further peripheral veins are not well evaluated for reflux using Valsalva's. Distal veins are then better evaluated using release of distal compression in a standing patient.

VALVE COUNT
The deep venous valves increase craniocaudally, and are rarely found above inguinal ligament i.e., in the iliac vein. Approximately 5 (range being 2-9) valves are noted in

between inguinal ligament and popliteal fossa. Below the popliteal vein level, there are numerous valves in tibial and peroneal veins, approximately at 2 cm intervals.[5,6,7]

The valves in popliteal vein ought to be competent for the calf muscle pump to be effective.

GSV trunk usually has at least 6 valves, and the SSV usually has 7-10 valves.[7] The medial calf and thigh perforators have 1-3 valves.[7]

Abnormalities relating to the valve could be:
- Absence of valves
- Dysfunction of valve due to degenerative changes
- Dysfunctional valve following recanalization of occlusive thrombus.
- Valve does not have a chance to function due to chronic venous obstruction

MUSCLE PUMPS

Muscle pumps involve muscle groups constrained by deep fascia. During the muscular contraction, the pressures within these compartments rise significantly, sufficient enough to eject venous blood out of the capacitance venous pools within them. The three muscle pumps available to the lower extremity are the thigh, calf and ankle. Together these 3 pumps are responsible for 90 % of the venous return from lower extremity, most important being the calf muscle pump.[6,8,9]

Let's see what happened when the muscle pumps contract. (see sketch 2.7).

Sketch 2.7. Musculovenous pump hemodynamics.

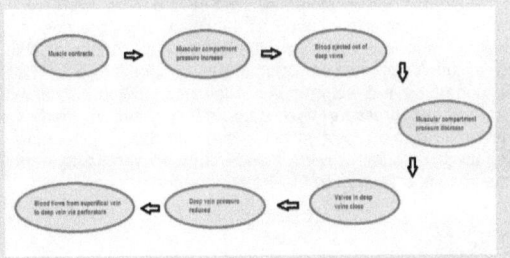

Contraction leads to high pressure within the muscle compartment. This then causes ejection of blood from deep veins of these compartments. The pressure then drops in these compartments. Subsequently the deep veins valves close, preventing retrograde flow. This post contraction reduction of deep venous pressure allows flow of blood from superficial venous system to deep venous system through the way of perforators.[6] (see chart 2.8).

Chart 2.8. Muscle compartment physiology

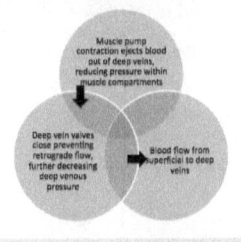

The muscle pump may fail due to musculo-fascial weakness, loss of joint motion or outflow obstruction.

The entire mechanism when normally operating tends to decrease the lower extremity venous pressure from 100 mmHg to 22 mmHg within 7 to 12 steps, while walking [10]. The calf muscle pump having the largest capacitance ejects 40 to 60 % of venous volume per contraction. [9,11] The venous blood is directed cranially towards iliofemoral veins. The venous pressure thus gets reduced, which then is reinforced by closure of valves, preventing reflux, generating negative pressure, drawing blood into deep venous system from the superficial veins via the perforators.

Primary valvular incompetence

Incompetence here is secondary to venous wall dilatation, the cause of which is unknown. There however are structural and/or biochemical changes within the venous wall, which leads to weak wall, venous dilatation, that then prevents coaptation of valve leaflets, thereby leading to reflux.[14] **The venous wall changes precede the reflux.**[11]

The histologic changes within the venous may be multifocal, and may vary in appearance at different locations, the characteristic changes being loss of elastic fibers, thickening of collagen fibers and disorganized muscle layer.[15,6]

The multi-centricity of primary valvular incompetence can be seen simultaneously in different venous segments which do not necessarily have to be in continuity.[15] These abnormalities are seen involving GSV, its tributaries and perforators.

Cause of these histological wall changed have been unclear and several mechanisms including inhibition of programmed cell death, enzyme activity changes, hypoxia mediated endothelial changes, etc. have been proposed.[6]

Secondary valvular incompetence

Reflux is the culprit here as well, but the cause of reflux is more or less a known event, such as post-thrombotic damage of valves. Recanalization of thrombosed venous lumen is rarely complete, and often there are strands of residual thrombi adherent to the vein wall, which over the course of time get fibrosed. If these residual thrombi happened to be closer to the attachment sites of valve leaflets, the fibrotic process engulf the leaflets, and restrict their motion, or the thrombus could cause endothelial erosion.[16] Thrombus alone is not the only entity which can push the vein through this route. Venous obstruction may be caused by a tumor, could be surgical or traumatic.

Ambulatory venous hypertension and Chronic venous insufficiency (CVI)

Whatever the cause of valve damage or dysfunction, the net result would is abnormal reflux. Reflux is seen in both primary and secondary valvular incompetence. This reflux raises the venous pressure in the post contraction relaxation phase within the deep veins. In the initial stages, the muscle pump tries to compensate for this reflux and prevent symptoms of insufficiency, or in fact delay the onset of clinical symptoms. [12,13,21] **That's the role of effective muscle pump in temporarily controlling the developing problem.** One may safely assume that the presence of pump dysfunction in presence of venous reflux from other cause may potentiate the progression of CVI. Subsequently, however over time the pressure remains persistently elevated and is overwhelming for the pump to compensate, resulting in ambulatory venous hypertension. Obviously, the development of this hypertension is expected to be slower in primary venous incompetence as compared to secondary incompetence, due to mechanical reasons present in the latter. The persistently elevated pressures in calf cause blood to be refluxed from deep venous system into superficial system, or at least inadequate emptying of superficial veins (see chart 2.9). There, in effect, is venous pooling in venous system of lower extremity. This leads to extravasation of intravascular contents into the adjoining interstitial space. The failure to reduce venous pressure with exercise is called Ambulatory venous hypertension. The clinical manifestations resulting from this venous hypertension are encompassed in the term Chronic Venous insufficiency (CVI).

The above discussion provides one more important clinical implication, which is the requirement to encompass

Chart 2.9. Chronic venous insufficiency hemodynamics

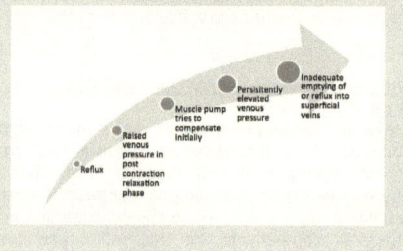

calf muscle pump treatment in the camp of CVI management. This may be addressed with exercise program or other measures.

Having reached at the stage of chronic venous insufficiency from the venous hypertension, we will try to see how this pathophysiology gives us the clinical picture we expect to see in our patients.

Ambulatory venous pressure (AVP) can be measured in a dorsal foot vein, after 10 tip toe maneuver, using 21 gauge needle.[10,17] Following the maneuver, the hydrostatic pressure restores after a mean time of 31 seconds.[11] Increased AVP is associated with 90% venous refill time of < 20 seconds.[17] The venous refill time decreases in presence of pathological reflux, and therefore the AVP increases. The venous outflow obstruction also raises AVP, initially during muscle contraction, and then in resting state as well.

There is linear relationship between ulcer incidence and AVP increase above 30 mmHg.

Plethysmography can measure volume changes in the limb. Rapid reflux, which is venous filling > 7 mL/sec are associated with high incidence of ulceration.[11,18]

The ejection fraction (EF) of calf muscle pump is a measure of its ability to eject blood, and is measured by calculating volume of blood ejected in one tip toe maneuver as percentage of resting venous volume.[19] In healthy subjects calf muscle pump EF is approximately 65 % and the thigh muscle pump EF is 15 %.

The threshold value for EF at which calf muscle pump may be described as dysfunctional range from 42-62 %, however healthy individuals may be seen falling in this range, thereby rendering this range as not the absolute range for diagnosis.[21]

Venous filling index (VFI)[20] = 90% of venous volume / time required to fill 90% of venous volume after resuming upright position

Normal VFI < 2 mL/s. This is increased in reflux and muscle pump dysfunction.

The skin and subcutaneous manifestations of CVI include edema, pigmentation, fibrosis and ulceration.

The common belief has been that venous stasis, in combination with low oxygen content of venous blood results in breakdown of overlying skin. Counterintuitive to this belief, it has been shown that the venous blood draining the ulcers have high oxygen content, and the flow through the ulcer bed is rapid. [22,23] Several other suggested theories include opening of AV fistula in response to increased venous pressure, exudation of fluid, increased interstitial fluid protein content, and inflammatory mechanisms.[11]

An update on CVI induced inflammatory processes can be found in several articles. [24,26]

REFERENCES

1. Pittaluga, P. et al. Influence on Chronic Venous Insufficiency of Primary Absence of the Great Saphenous Vein in the Saphenous Compartment at the Thigh. Journal of Vascular Surgery: Venous and Lymphatic Disorders , Volume 1 , Issue 1 , 101
2. Spencer, L. et al. Klippel-Trenaunay Syndrome and Left Iliac Vein Agenesis. EJVES Extra , Volume 13 , Issue 3 , 50 - 51
3. Herman J, Musil D. Klippel-Trénaunay syndrome associated with great saphenous vein aplasia. Phlebology. 2010 Feb;25(1):35-7. doi: 10.1258/phleb.2009.008079.
4. van Bemmelen PS, Beach K, Bedford G, Strandness DE, Jr. The Mechanism of Venous Valve Closure: It's Relationship to the Velocity of Reverse Flow. *Arch Surg.* 990;125(5):617-619
5. Negus D. The surgical anatomy of the veins of the lower limb. In: Dodd H, Cockett FB, eds. The Pathology and Surgery of the Veins of the Lower Limb. 2nd ed. Edinburgh: Churchill Livingstone; 1976:18–49.
6. Meissner MH. Lower extremity venous anatomy. Semin Intervent Radiol 2005; 22:147–156.
7. Mozes G, Carmichael SW, Gloviczki P. Development and anatomy of the venous system. In: Gloviczki P, Yao JST, eds. Handbook of Venous Disorders: Guidelines of the American Venous Forum. 2nd ed. London: Arnold; 2001:11–24

8. Goldman MP, Fronek A. Anatomy and pathophysiology of varicose veins. J Dermatol Surg Oncol 1989;15:138–145
9. Ludbrook J. The musculovenous pumps of the human lower limb. Am Heart J 1966;71:635–641
10. Pollack AA, Wood EH. Venous pressure in the saphenous vein at the ankle in man during exercise and changes in posture. J Appl Physiol 1949;1:649-62.
11. Meissner, Mark H. et al. The hemodynamics and diagnosis of venous disease. J Vasc Surg 2007; 46(6): S4 - S24
12. Padberg FT, Jr., Johnston MV, Sisto SA. Structured exercise improves calf muscle pump function in chronic venous insufficiency: a randomized trial. J Vasc Surg 2004;39:79-87.
13. Plate G, Brudin L, Eklof B, Jensen R, Ohlin P. Congenital vein valve aplasia. World J Surg 1986;10:929-34.
14. Alexander CJ. The theoretical basis of varicose vein formation. Med J Aust 1972;1:258-61.
15. Labropoulos N, Giannoukas AD, Delis K, et al. Where does venous reflux start? J Vasc Surg 1997;26:736–742
16. Budd TW, Meenaghan MA, Wirth J, Taheri SA. Histopathology of veins and venous valves of patients with venous insufficiency syndrome: ultrastructure. J Med 1990;21:181–199
17. Nicolaides AN, Hussein MK, Szendro G, Christopoulos D, Vasdekis S, Clarke H. The relationship of venous ulceration with ambulatory venous pressure measurements. J Vasc Surg 1993;17:414-9.
18. Christopoulos DG, Nicolaides AN, Szendro G, Irvine AT, Bull ML, Eastcott HH. Air-plethysmography and the effect of elastic compression on venous hemodynamics of the leg. J Vasc Surg 1987;5:148-59.
19. Welkie JF, Comerota AJ, Katz ML, Aldridge SC, Kerr RP, White JV.Hemodynamic deterioration in chronic venous disease. J Vasc Surg 1992;16:733-40.

20. Christopoulos D, Nicolaides AN, Szendro G. Venous reflux: quantification and correlation with the clinical severity of chronic venous disease. Br J Surg 1988;75:352-6.
21. Katherine J. Williams, Olufemi Ayekoloye, Hayley M. Moore, Alun H. Davies, The calf muscle pump revisited, Journal of Vascular Surgery: Venous and Lymphatic Disorders 2014; 2(3): 329-334.
22. Clarke GH, Vasdekis SN, Hobbs JT, Nicolaides AN. Venous wall function in the pathogenesis of varicose veins. Surgery 1992;111: 402-8.
23. Hopkins NF, Spinks TJ, Rhodes CG, Ranicar AS, Jamieson CW. Positron emission tomography in venous ulceration and liposclerosis:study of regional tissue function. Br Med J (Clin Res Ed) 1983 Jan 29;286:333-6
24. Coleridge Smith PD. Update on chronic-venous-insufficiency-induced inflammatory processes. Angiology 2001;52 (Suppl 1):S35-S42.
25. Nicos Labropoulos, Jay Tiongson, Landon Pryor, Apostolos K Tassiopoulos, Steven S Kang, M Ashraf Mansour, William H Baker, Definition of venous reflux in lower-extremity veins, Journal of Vascular Surgery, 2003; 38(4): 793-798
26. Meissner MH et al. Primary chronic venous disorders. J Vasc Surg. 2007 Dec;46 Suppl S:54S-67S

Chapter 3

CLINICAL PRESENTATION

Chapter facts to remember (see chart 3.1 – 3.3)

Chart 3.1. Facts to remember

Symptoms of CVI

- Leg pain or discomfort
- Calf muscle cramps
- Leg swelling
- Discoloration of legs
- Ulcer(s), recurrent ulcer(s), non healing ulcer(s).
- Dilated tortuous visible veins
- Itching
- Numbness, tingling
- Generalized fatigue
- Spontaneous bleeding
- No symptoms – incidentally found by self or health provider exam.

Terminology

- Telangiectasia: < 1mm dilated intradermal venules
- Reticular veins: 1-3 mm dilated subdermal veins
- Varicose: > 3mm dilated superficial veins

Diagnosis of varicose veins

- ✓ Patients complain
- ✓ Physical signs
- ✓ Diagnostic imaging (color Doppler)

Chart 3.2. Facts to remember

Risk factors – modifiable
- Obesity
- Lifestyle
- Smoking

Risk factor for unhealed ulcer(s)
- Age > 60 years
- Extensive lipodermatosclerosis
- Prior history of ulceration.

Risk factors – non-modifiable
- Advancing age
- Family history of venous disease
- History of DVT

Risk factor for recurrence of ulcer(s)
- first episode ≥ 2 years
- incompetence of venous systems.

Chart 3.3. Facts to remember

Other causes that can give leg swelling besides CVI

- Deep vein thrombosis
- Congestive heart failure
- Renal failure
- Lymphatic obstruction
- Bakers cyst, ruptured

There is wide spectrum of clinical presentation of this health condition. It has never ceased to amaze us the extent to which this venous disease can progress, if not addressed. In order to prevent the extreme clinical picture, earlier identification of this disease condition is crucial.

The most common single presentation that we have seen in our clinical practice is leg pain. This may or may not be associated with other signs and symptoms, which we discuss later. Other leading presentations can be leg swelling, visible tortuous veins in lower extremities, discoloration of leg and feet, leg cramps, etc. The extreme and most uncomfortable of these is leg ulceration, especially the non-healing ulcers.

Although we are not sure of the popularity of CEAP classification in various parts of the world, it provides a systematic approach to identify and describe the clinical picture of individual patient, but does not estimate severity of disease, and is not designed to measure changes in patient's condition.[1]

The Venous severity scores assess the severity, and Quality of life scores assess outcomes.[3]

LEG PAIN

Patients, at their initial presentation, often complain of leg pain, which is described as dull aching, progressive during the day, and is the most at bedtime. Lying down supine makes them feel better, and a nighttime sleep provides relief by morning. Some are not so fortunate, and are kept awake by the pain. By the time these patients present, they already have tried several pain relieving medications, which may have worked in the beginning, but do not provide symptomatic relief any more. In the past, this condition was associated with professions requiring long hours of erect posture, for example, traffic policemen and bus conductors. But as we saw in the pathophysiology chapter, erect posture may not be the only cause, although it may be a precipitating factor. Leg pain or specifically calf pain is usually described as dull aching, non- radiating, of variable intensity. Patients provide differing alleviating and aggravating factors for leg pain, but by the time medical help is sought, there are few, if any alleviating factors. Pain may also be localized to a specific region, for example, ulcerated region or thrombosed superficial vein.

CALF CRAMPS
Leg cramps are often mistaken as calf pain, the history of which may be elicited by differing descriptions in languages best understood by patient.

DISCOLORATION / PIGMENTATION
Discoloration involves the medial ankle initially, and then subsequently progresses to involve foot and leg above ankle. Patients often describe this as progressive and increasing in extent as well as intensity. Some individuals may not have noticed this at all, and in them it is probably best appreciated by the health care provider, family members or friends. The brown or bluish grey pigmentation is derived from breakdown of extravasated red blood cells in the dermis, which provides hemosiderin deposition (see image 3.4). This may be associated with thick coarse skin at firm indurated area, described as lipodermatosclerosis, which is fibrosing panniculitis of subcutaneous tissue. This again is usually seen initially at medial ankle and then progresses to involve leg above the ankles.

LEG SWELLING
Leg swelling is similar to the leg pain. It is progressive in time course, increasing through the day, and is described the most at bedtime. Initially the swelling may just be around the ankle, but later progresses to involve the calf region as well (see image 3.5). It may then persist throughout the day. We have seen patients with varicose veins, having complain of leg swelling even when they get up in the morning, and certainly in those conditions other causes of leg swelling also need to be considered which may or may not be associated with CVI. But CVI by itself can also do that, especially in obese population. The commonest description of swelling described by a patient is that which worsens on standing,

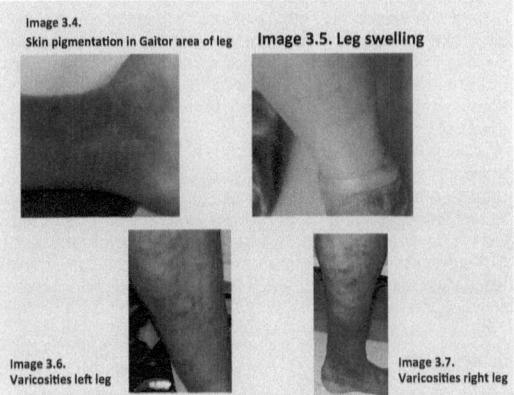

Image 3.4.
Skin pigmentation in Gaitor area of leg

Image 3.5. Leg swelling

Image 3.6.
Varicosities left leg

Image 3.7.
Varicosities right leg

and improves on leg elevation. It's not surprising to know that some patients describe using pillows beneath the legs/ankles to elevate the leg while supine, and sometimes in sitting position as well. Women may describe worsening of symptoms during pregnancy or even during menses, which is likely related to increased fluid volume and/or estrogen.

DILATED TORTOUS VEINS

Varicosities, in simple terms, described as tortuous and swollen veins is the commonest accompanying complain, but patients presenting with the only intention of getting those treated (i.e. having no other symptoms) for cosmetic reasons, although relatively a fewer percentage, are tending to show early in disease course (see image 3.6 and 3.7). Varicosities are common incidental findings on a physical exam performed for different reason. The size of externally visible varicosities does not provide real picture of what's going on inside, and up to one half of patients may be asymptomatic.[4] On the other hand, symptomatic patient may not have visible tortuous veins on the outside.

ULCER (New, recurrent, or non-healing)

Leg ulceration is the extreme presentation of this spectrum of disease. But understanding them helps us dealing with them. Venous ulcers have typical locations, along the medial aspect of mid to lower leg, described by some as gaiter area (extending from calf muscles where they become prominent posteriorly, up to below the malleoli level inferiorly) (see images 3.8 and 3.9). Gaiters are garments worn over the shoe and lower pants, and used primarily as personal protective equipment. Foot and above knee ulcers should virtually rule out venous ulcers, although extension of above ankle ulcers can be seen into the foot. But ulcers involving only the dorsal foot or posterior leg are less frequent.

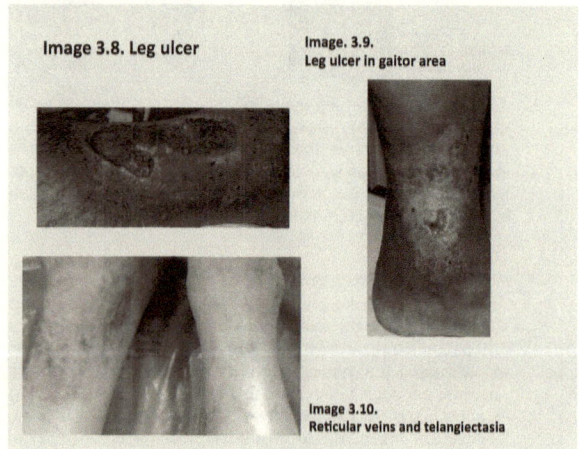

Image 3.8. Leg ulcer

Image. 3.9. Leg ulcer in gaitor area

Image 3.10. Reticular veins and telangiectasia

At often times, the patient may describe that the ulcers healed in the past, but recur and do not heal anymore. Apart from the discomfort they provide, the ulcers are potential route for infections. Approximately 40 % of ulcers remain unhealed in < 1 year. The risk factor for unhealed ulcers are age > 60, extensive lipodermatosclerosis, and prior history of ulceration.[5] The risk factor for recurrence include first episode ≥ 2 years, and incompetence of venous systems.

Uncontrolled diabetes mellitus may also impact the healing of ulcers. No statistical significance has been found in terms of differences in right or left limb involvement.

OTHER SYMPTOMS

Itching, numbness and tingling, and generalized fatigue are other symptomatic complains provided by patients. In some, stasis dermatitis may be the initial presentation of disease, which is characterized by dry, scaly and itchy skin, with some crusting and erythema. Patients repeated scratching marks may be identified on skin, with some areas of skin breakdown.

Rarely patient with known disease may present with bleeding from varicosities, particularly induced by trauma over the site of varicosities. This may possibly be the only condition when you may have to act emergently to manage these patients.

Approximately 20 % of symptomatic patients have no clinical sigins.[4] Duplex exam is helpful is demonstrating venous reflux in these patients.

The fact that there is varied presentation of this disease, which may be associated with other health conditions; a detailed physical exam should be performed, addressing the venous aspect, as well as arterial and neurological assessment of the limb. Additionally, needless to mention general health of patient needs to be addressed too. For example, obesity, diabetes mellitus, and lifestyle modification may be have to be part of management tools.

Several less than 1 mm dilated intradermal venules termed as Telangiectasia may be seen.[2] Dilated and tortuous subdermal veins 1-3 mm in diameter represent reticular veins.² (see image 3.10) Dilated and tortuous subcutaneous veins, greater than 3 mm diameter are the varicose veins, which could be any vein(s) of the superficial venous system.²

Some of the risk factors for CVI are also associated with other health conditions, particularly the coronary or peripheral arterial disease, and so it's recommended that the patients, particularly with the known risk factors, be evaluated for those diseases as well.

A large nationwide epidemiological survey conducted in Italy in 2003 enrolled > 5000 individuals, who were evaluated clinically and with lower extremity ultrasound exam. Results from this study provides a snap shot of CVD pattern prevailing in population at large, although these may not be a representation of global population at large.[4]

Approximately 20 % of population demonstrated truncal varicosities. Incidence increases with age, BMI and number of pregnancies. Statistical significance exists between BMI or family history of CVD and frequency of CVD. 80 % of individuals having symptomatic complains but having no signs of CVI, did not demonstrate reflux. The frequency of reflux increased with the severity of visible signs of disease.

CEAP CLASSIFICATION

CEAP classification was developed in 1994 by American Venous Forum, which was later revised in 2004. CEAP classification is a consensus document, which is adopted worldwide to communicate CVD status effectively. It is composed of clinical manifestations (C), etiologic factors (E), anatomic distribution of disease (A), and underlying pathophysiologic findings (P).[2] It provides a systematic and uniform evaluation of venous disease

The "C" component i.e., clinical manifestations of CVD are grouped and sub grouped into:

C_0: No visible or palpable signs of venous disease.
C_1: Telangiectasia's or reticular signs.
C_2: Varicose veins (distinguished from reticular veins by a diameter of 3mm or more).
C_3: Edema.
C_{4a}: Pigmentation or eczema.
C_{4b}: Lipodermatosclerosis or atrophie blanche.
C_5: Healed venous ulcer.
C_6: Active venous ulcer.
S: Symptomatic, includes, ache, pain, tightness, skin irritation, heaviness and muscle cramps, and other complains attributable to venous dysfunction.
A: Asymptomatic.

"E" Etiologic classification

Ec: Congenital
Ep: Primary
Es: Secondary (post thrombotic or tumor compression)
En: No venous cause identified.

"A" Anatomic classification

As: superficial veins
Ap: perforator veins
Ad: deep veins
An: no venous location identified

"P" Pathophysiologic classification

Basic CEAP
Pr: reflux
Po: obstruction
Pr,o: reflux and obstruction
Pn: no venous pathophysiology identifiable

Advanced CEAP: Adds any of 18 named venous segments to locate venous pathology.

Superficial veins
Telangiectasia's or reticular veins
Great saphenous vein above knee
Great saphenous vein below knee
Small saphenous vein
Nonsaphenous veins

Deep veins
Inferior vena cava
Common iliac vein
Internal iliac vein
External iliac vein
Pelvic: gonadal, broad ligament veins, other
Common femoral vein
Deep femoral vein
Femoral vein
Popliteal vein
Crural: anterior tibial, posterior tibial, peroneal veins (all paired)
Muscular: gastrocnemial, soleal veins, other.

Perforating veins:
Thigh
Calf

The increase in medial calf perforating veins number and their diameter, particularly those permitting bidirectional flows, is associated with deteriorating CVI and the CEAP grade.[6]
Advanced CEAP disease may also be associated with a considerable increase in superficial and deep venous reflux, which may encompass short saphenous vein as well.

Venous severity scoring system[3]

2 scores are proposed:

1. Venous clinical severity score (VCSS): 9 clinical characteristics of CVD are graded from 0 to 3 (absent, mild, moderate, severe).
2. Venous segmental disease score (VSDS): assesses 11 venous segments for reflux and/or obstruction.

Here, we discuss VCSS. The VSDS, after long work was still arbitrary, and a discussion on this topic, and reasons why further modifications are recommended are discussed by Rutherford et al.[3]

VCSS

(I) **Pain :**
   Absent, 0: None
   Mild, 1: Occasional, not restricting activity or requiring analgesics
   Moderate, 2: Daily, moderate activity limitation, occasional analgesics
   Severe, 3: Daily, severe limiting activities or requiring regular use of analgesics

(II) **Varicose veins** (must be > 4-mm diameter to qualify so that differentiation is ensured between C1 and C2 venous pathology):
   Absent, 0: None
   Mild, 1: Few, scattered: branch varicose veins.
   Moderate, 2: Multiple: greater saphenous varicose veins confined to calf or thigh.
   Severe, 3: Extensive: Thigh *and* calf or greater and shorter saphenous distribution.

(III) **Venous edema** (Presumes venous origin by characteristics (e.g., Brawny [not pitting or spongy] edema), with significant effect of standing/limb elevation and/or other clinical evidence of venous etiology (i.e., varicose veins, history of DVT). Edema must be regular finding

(e.g., daily occurrence). Occasional or mild edema does not qualify.)
    Absent, 0: None.
    Mild, 1: Evening ankle edema only
    Moderate, 2 Afternoon edema, above ankle
    Severe, 3: Morning edema above ankle and requiring activity change, elevation.

(IV) **Skin pigmentation** (Focal pigmentation over varicose veins does not qualify):
    Absent, 0: None or focal, low intensity (tan).
    Mild, 1: Diffuse, but limited in area and old (brown)
    Moderate, 2 Diffuse over most of gaiter distribution (lower 1/3) *or* recent pigmentation (purple)
    Severe, 3: Wider distribution (above lower 1/3) *and* recent pigmentation

(V) **Inflammation**
    Absent, 0: None.
    Mild, 1: Mild cellulitis, limited to marginal area around ulcer
    Moderate, 2: Moderate cellulitis, involves most of gaiter area (lower 1/3)
    Severe, 3: Severe cellulitis (lower 1/3 and above) or significant venous eczema

(VI) **Induration**
    Absent, 0: None.
    Mild, 1: Focal, circummalleolar (< 5 cm)
    Moderate, 2: Medial or lateral, less than lower third of leg
    Severe, 3: Entire lower third of leg or more

(VII) **Number of active ulcers**
    Absent, 0: 0
    Mild, 1: 1
    Moderate, 2: 2
    Severe, 3: > 2

(VIII) <u>Active ulceration, duration</u>
Absent, 0: None
Mild, 1: < 3 months
Moderate, 2: > 3 months, < 1 year
Severe, 3: Not healed > 1 year.

(IX) ***Active ulcer, size*** (Largest dimension/diameter of largest ulcer)
Absent, 0: None
Mild, 1: < 2 cm diameter
Moderate, 2: 2-6 cm diameter
Severe, 3: > 6 cm diameter

(X) ***Compressive therapy*** (Sliding scale to adjust for background differences in use of compressive therapy):
Absent, 0: Not used or not compliant
Mild, 1 Intermittent use of stockings
Moderate, 2: Wears elastic stockings most days
Severe, 3: Full compliance: stockings + elevation

CLINICAL RELEVANCE

Although majority of these individual questions which comprise severity scoring may change over time following treatment, the scoring on ulceration changes the most, but still do not contribute significantly to the overall score.[7] Lattimer et al used VCSS and Aberdeen varicose vein questionnaire (AVVQ) to quantify effects of treatment. In their prospective study, the median interquartile VCSS and AVVQ scores improved following treatment. Pain, edema and extent of varicosities i.e., questions 1-3 were most contributory to overall score. VCSS had greater correlation with AVVQ in this study. Timing of obtaining the post procedure scoring is also important, since invariably you find worsening of score in immediate post-operative period. Beyond 3 weeks would be appropriate time to evaluate. However, some components of the scoring system, for e.g., induration, may take more than 3 months to improve, and component like pigmentation, even longer.

REFERENCES:

1. Meissner, Mark H. et al. The hemodynamics and diagnosis of venous disease. J Vasc Surg 2007; 46(6): S4 - S24
2. Eklof B, Rutherford RB, Bergan JJ, Carpentier PH, Gloviczki P, Kistner RL, et al. Revision of the CEAP classification for chronic venous disorders: consensus statement. J Vasc Surg 2004;40:1248-52.
3. Rutherford RB, Padberg FT, Comerota AJ, Kistner RL, Meissner MH, Moneta GL. Venous severity scoring: an adjunct to venous outcome assessment. J Vasc Surg 2000;31:1307-12.
4. Chiesa R, Marone EM, Limoni C, et al. Chronic venous disorders: correlation between visible signs, symptoms, and presence of functional disease. J Vasc Surg 2007; 46:322.
5. Abbade LP, Lastória S, Rollo Hde A. Venous ulcer: clinical characteristics and risk factors. Int J Dermatol 2011; 50:405-411.
6. Stuart WP et al. The relationship between the number, competence, and diameter of medial calf perforating veins and the clinical status in healthy subjects and patients with lower-limb venous disease. J Vasc Surg 2000;32:138-43.
7. C R Lattimer, E Kalodiki, M Azzam and G Geroulakos. Responsiveness of individual questions from the venous clinical severity score and the Aberdeen varicose vein questionnaire. J Vasc Surg 2012; 55(1):298–299

Chapter 4

ULTRASOUND IMAGING

Chapter facts to remember (see chart 4.1 – 4.3)

Chart 4.1. Facts to remember

Deep veins to be evaluated by US

- IVC
- Common iliac vein
- External iliac vein
- Common femoral vein
- Femoral vein (SFV)
- Profunda (deep femoral)
- Popliteal – above knee
- Popliteal – below knee
- Posterior tibial veins (paired)
- Peroneal veins (paired)
- Anterior tibial veins (paired)

US format for evaluation of lower extremity deep veins for DVT

B- Mode -
- Compressibility of lumen
- Lumen echogenicity / presence of thrombus

Color mode -
- Color flow –present/ absent
- Reflux on valsalvas

Duplex mode -
- Phasic variation with respiration.
- Augmentation on distal compression
- Venous reflux (use valsalva's for femoropopliteal only)

Chart 4.2. Facts to remember

Superficial veins to be evaluated by US
- SFJ
- GSV
- Accessory GSV
- Collaterals of GSV
- SSV

US evaluation specifics to GSV (and SSV)

- Presence / absence of certain segments
- Duplication
- Diameter (as a whole or if focally increased or decreased)
- Tortuosity (which can hamper advancement of laser fiber).
- Fusiform dilatation (can be obstacle for fiber advancement – gentle external pressure can straighten the lumen path, and then the fiber can be advanced under US guidance).

US format for evaluation of Superficial veins (including SF junction and SP junction)

B Mode:
- Compressibility of lumen
- Luminal echogenicity – anechoic or presence of thrombus

Color mode -
- Color flow
- Reflux

Duplex mode -
- Augmentation
- Venous reflux on valsalvas

Chart 4.3. Facts to remember

Ultrasound transducer's required for lower extremity venous imaging
- 3-5 Mhz
- 10-12 Mhz
- 5-7 Mhz (optional)

US format for evaluation of Perforators
Patency of lumen
Presence of color flow
Reflux of color flow on distal compression

MANEUVRE FOR ELICITING VENOUS REFLUX

- After a quick compression, release the extremity
- Antegrade flow is followed by a retrograde flow
- If this retrograde flow persists for longer duration than normal, pathological reflux is documented.
- Otherwise, the reflux is labelled physiological reflux.

INTRODUCTION

As in many other disease conditions, Ultrasound (US) imaging has created its impact in the field of lower extremity venous diseases, particularly the deep venous thrombosis and chronic venous insufficiency. In this chapter we will discuss the machinery required, patient positioning, scanning technique, various criteria's and will have some images to look at.

INDICATIONS/ROLE OF US

1. Diagnostic – to diagnose the presence and extent of chronic venous insufficiency, recurrence of disease, and to exclude deep vein thrombosis.
2. Interventional – US is an essential component in management of varicose veins, as it helps plan the therapeutic endovenous procedure, and also serves as the mapping guide during the endovenous laser procedure.
3.

MACHINERY

Unit : A color doppler unit is required for this purpose. A standalone unit or portable unit may serve this purpose. The key point is comfortness of the operator to use whichever machine is incorporated for this purpose.

Transducers : A convex abdominal prone (3-5 MHz frequency), and Linear high frequency probe (10-12 MHz) is required with the unit.

PATIENT POSITIONING

Patient may be scanned in supine, sitting or standing (upright) positions. For diagnostic purposes one may have to scan in standing position, since the gravitational effect is manifested and the abnormality in vein physiology becomes evident. By international consensus, the diagnostic US exam is performed in upright position.

However, for the mapping purposes there are different preferences. At most of the times, for mapping purposes only (once diagnosis has been established), we have preferred scanning in supine position, since that's the position patient would be in during the procedure. This gives a fair idea of how the veins would look like when intervention is being performed. But if there is a discrepancy between diagnostic scan and mapping scan performed prior to the procedure, we have preferred scanning in upright position and mark accordingly.

It must be kept in mind though the criteria for reflux are based on upright positions, as described later in this chapter.

ROOM ENVIRONMENT

Ultrasound exam should be performed in an environment that is comfortable to the patient. Extremes of temperature may alter the adrenergic impulses and skin circulation, leading to erroneous results. A cool room may provide false positive results. A systemic illness or hypovolemia may lead to lack of venous distension and thereby provide false-negative results.[9]

MACHINE SETTINGS

Most of the settings in current machines come as presets and a "Venous" preset for extremity may be selected. However, with different patients, the color gain settings and PRF (Pulse Repetition frequency) may have to be set low enough for venous signals.

ULTRASOUND TOOLS AVAILABLE

B-Mode : used to evaluate lumen and compressibility.

Color-mode : to see presence of color flow and reflux.

Duplex-mode :
- Spectral waveform to document reflux.
- Phasic variation to evaluate venous system central to the area being scanned.
- Augmentation of flow on distal compression to document patency of lumen peripheral to the area being scanned, as well as demonstrating reflux in popliteal and calf veins.

ULTRASOUND TECHNIQUE AND PROTOCOL

The Ultrasound exam of lower extremity venous system includes the B- mode, Color mode and Duplex mode exam.

IVC and Iliac veins

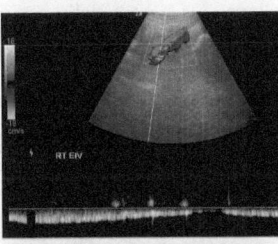

4.4 Image. Spectral waveform and color flow in a normal external iliac vein

In our practice, we start ultrasound scanning with the inferior vena cava (IVC) and the iliac veins, using the convex transducer. This helps us rule out any abdominal pathology which may be the cause of patient's symptoms or may directly or indirectly affect management of patient. Examples of these abdominal pathologies are thrombosed IVC and / or iliac veins, abdominal / pelvis mass compressing the veins, extrinsic hematoma, lymph nodes, aneurysm, etc.

The IVC and iliac veins are evaluated first in transverse section and then in longitudinal section, for lumen, presence of color flow, and spectral waveform. The waveform is a representative of what's happening centrally in venous system, and the phasic variation in these veins should be identified, with the exceptions being patient in heart failure (See image 4.4). In presence of proximal occlusion (or central occlusion), monophasic waveform is appreciated.

Transducer switch

Once the IVC and iliac veins have been evaluated, the transducer may be switched from convex abdominal to linear high frequency probe. In patients with grossly edematous or enlarged swollen lower extremities, we have even performed the lower extremity venous exam using the convex abdominal transducer which provides advantage of evaluating deeper structures. In our set up we had availability of an endocavitary transducer which was of intermediate frequency between the convex abdominal and the high frequency. This enables visualization of vein and adjoining soft tissue structures located at intermediate depth from the skin.

Deep venous system

In the lower extremity, we prefer to start scanning with deep venous system, to rule out deep vein thrombosis and to evaluate presence of reflux. The deep veins described in chapter of anatomy are then evaluated for lumen, diameter, compressibility, color flow, spectral waveform – phasic variation, and augmentation of flow on distal compression (see image 4.5).

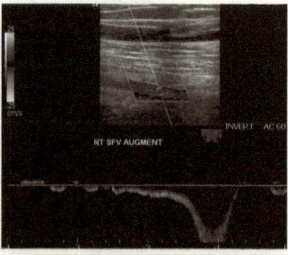

4.5 Image. Augmentation noted in spectral waveform through a deep vein

The popliteal vein may have to be scanned in prone position if not evaluated in ipsilateral supine oblique position. The paired posterior tibial veins and peroneal veins are evaluated for color flow and compressibility (see images 4.6).

Presence of deep vein thrombosis essentially leaves the superficial venous system as the alternative for venous drainage in lower extremity. This then may be the cause of patient's symptoms but may also preclude performing endovenous laser to keep the sole venous drainage channel open.

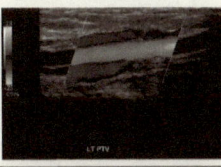

4.6 Image. Normal paired posterior tibial veins accompanying the posterior tibial artery in leg.

Significance of deep venous reflux

It's important to evaluate the presence of deep venous reflux, since 6% of CVI patients could have isolated deep venous reflux, in addition to the combined scenarios where superficial and/or perforator system could also be involved.[11] With the treatment of superficial venous reflux, most of the deep venous reflux disappears.[12] However, this response may be influenced by etiology of this reflux, which may be primary (structural abnormalities in venous wall and/or valves, agenesis of valves), or secondary (post deep vein thrombosis). A safe and effective treatment for deep venous reflux is yet to be proven, although deep reconstructive surgeries (for example, valvuloplasty, transposition, transplantation, neovalve, etc) have been attempted wordlwide.[13] Persistence of deep vein reflux presumably poses a risk for recurrence of varicose as well as venous ulcers, even after endovenous laser of superficial venous system.

Attention should be paid to duplication of deep venous system, and possible reflux or thrombus involving the duplicated segment of vein. Pitfalls of venous duplex imaging include compressibility evaluation in adductor canal region, however the patency of that vein segment may then be evaluated by color mode.

Superficial venous system
Having evaluated the deep venous system, we then evaluate superficial venous system. We usually start with locating the SFJ. Then we proceed down to rest of the superficial venous system.

Superficial venous system- SFJ
The confluence of veins at SFJ is localized on ultrasound in longitudinal section. Patency of the SFJ is established by demonstrating compressibility of venous lumen in a transverse scanning plane. SFJ dynamics is then evaluated at rest and during Valsalva's, using two means – color flow and duplex. The color flow images show patency of veins across the junction as well as change in color indicating reflux. Similarly duplex exam is performed and spectral waveform obtained at rest and Valsalva's maneuver. Note that physiological reflux is almost always seen, and it's the persistence of reflux beyond 0.5 seconds is diagnostic of incompetent SFJ.

Superficial venous system- GSV
Next, to be evaluated in superficial venous system is the GSV, which we evaluate from SFJ craniocaudally up to medial malleolus. GSV is evaluated for – its directional course, presence / absence in certain segments, anechoic lumen, compressibility, diameter, color flow and reflux, spectral waveform for reflux and augmentation on distal compression. We perform the exam first in transverse and then in longitudinal section.

The main saphenous trunk in the thigh is located within the saphenous compartment, which has been described as resembling the "Egyptian eye" (see sketch 4.7) on transverse ultrasound image. The GSV lumen represents the iris, superficial fascia representing upper eyelid and deep fascia representing lower eyelid.[10]

Alignment sign: Two saphenous eyes may be seen on transverse ultrasound scanning of upper third of thigh. This could be from GSV and AASV. AASV can be recognized by its location/alignment over the femoral artery and vein, but anterior and lateral to the GSV.

Superficial venous system- GSV tributaries
Next, we localize tributaries of GSV in thigh and in legs. They are evaluated for patency and reflux. Additionally they become important as route of access for endovenous procedure, if GSV is occluded, absent or for some part do not have reflux.

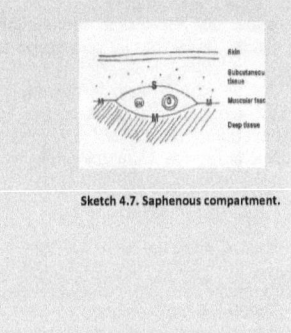

Sketch 4.7. Saphenous compartment.

Superficial venous system- SPJ, SSV and its tributaries
Following evaluation of GSV and its tributaries, we evaluate the SSV. While GSV incompetence is the dominant cause of venous CVI, approximately 13-20% of these patients have SSV incompetence.[7] The ablation results of GSV and SSV may differ due to two main factors : proximity of SSV to sural nerve, and the anatomical differences between SPJ and SFJ.[8] SSV evaluation may be performed in prone position or ipsilateral supine oblique position with leg flexed at knee. The SPJ is first localized, which usually is at or around the knee level in popliteal fossa. This is done

in longitudinal section. Once the junction is localized, color mode is used to evaluate color flow and reflux across the junction during rest and Valsalva's maneuver. Duplex mode is used to obtain spectral waveform during rest and Valsalva's or distal compression, thereby evaluating for presence/absence of reflux. The SSV, as is the GSV, is scanned first in transverse section followed by longitudinal section.

Three anatomic patterns of SSV drainage have been proposed by Gibson et al [8]:
Type A : into SPJ with no significant branches.
Type B: into SPJ with large cranial extension, the latter also called Giacomini vein.
Type C: No direct termination into deep vein, but continues as Giacomini vein above popliteal fossa.

The Giacomini vein of the short saphenous system can be considered analogous to the inferior epigastric vein in endovenous ablation of GSV. In type B, laser fiber may be positioned in the Giacomini vein so as to avoid deep vein.[8] Type C due to obvious reasons, will not have problem of DVT.

Next, the tributaries of SSV are evaluated.

Perforator venous system
A schematic pattern for perforator evaluation should be followed ensuring that the perforators described in chapter on anatomy are examined. The perforators are evaluated for diameter, reflux on color mode. The mapping scan performed prior to procedure is basically the same as described above. The course of superficial veins are marked using marker pen, as are the site of incompetent perforators. The typical locations to look for perforators are: medial, lateral and posterior leg, and medial distal one-third of thigh. Diameter is measured in B-mode, in transverse plane, and at the location where it pierces the fascia. Reflux is evaluated in color mode and duplex mode, along the long axis of

perforating vein, and by manual compressing of limb above and below the perforator level.

Ulcer

Special mention for ultrasound evaluation of venous system in limb having venous ulcer is required. Perforators adjoining the ulcer site need to be identified. The ulcer itself is painful, and care needs to be taken to keep it sterile. With the availability of sterile transducer cover and ultrasound jelly, ultrasound evaluation may be performed to look for underlying and/or adjoining incompetent perforators.

DIAGNOSTIC US FINDINGS

Diagnosing presence of venous reflux is the prime purpose of performing this exam. But besides this main purpose, there is some critical information we need to obtain. Foremost amongst them is to rule out presence of deep venous thrombosis. For the purposes of management, it's essential to know the level of venous reflux and presence of reflux in different vein segments.

DIAGNOSTIC US FINDINGS – DEEP VENOUS SYSTEM

(I) Deep venous thrombosis : The most important finding is to look for compressibility. This is performed using B-mode, in a transverse plane of the vein. Non compressibility is probably the most important of all the ultrasound findings which suggest thrombosis. Other things to look for are the caliber, luminal thrombus, color flow, phasic variation with respiration, and augmentation of flow on distal compression. Present of acute DVT dissuades one from performing varicose ablative procedure for preexisting varicosities, particularly because the latter being non emergent procedure, and also because anticoagulants may be used for treatment of DVT.

(II) As far as chronic DVT is concerned, we would consider other factors too. Say for example, if the DVT has been chronic, recanalized but recurring, then this pathway may not be the reliable one, and probably leaving the superficial venous system as the viable option for venous return may be the best available choice. However if there has been remote history of DVT which has remained recanalized with no recurrences, then dealing with the superficial venous system may be considered. Nevertheless, in these situations number of factors need to be considered, and each case may be different.

(III) Reflux in deep venous system. The reflux is evaluated in color mode as well as Duplex mode. The transducer plane is longitudinal, i.e. Along the venous lumen. Reflux is elicited by Valsalva' maneuver (in the common femoral and femoral veins), and by distal calf compression and release (in popliteal and calf veins). If present, its level should be documented.

DIAGNOSTIC US FINDINGS – SUPERFICIAL VENOUS SYSTEM

Evaluate for: Presence/absence of vein; compressible; patency/thrombosis; diameter; competency/reflux; anatomical variations in number and course of veins.

(I) Duplication of GSV in leg and/or thigh needs to be documented, as well as presence/ absence of reflux in them (see image 4.8). Needless to say, satisfaction of search with reflux identified on one of the duplicated GSV, and

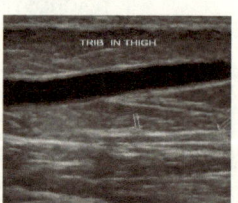

4.8 Image. Variant anatomy on ultrasound. Main GSV may be fibrosed (arrows) and there may be a prominent tributary in superficial plane that may serve as the main truncal vein.

not identifying other GSV could be potential cause of recurrence or failure of treatment.

(II) Diameter: Reflux is the only diagnostic imaging requirement of CVI. However, studies have shown diameter of GSV to be predictive of reflux in it. While we have not put that into practice and am not sure of its worldwide acceptance, it's interesting to note the figures provided by Navarro et al.[3]

GSV diameters highly predictive of incompetence (see image 4.9):
> 7.3 mm at SFJ,
> 6 mm at mid-thigh
> 4 mm at mid-calf

GSV diameters associated with lack of reflux:
< 5.5 mm at SFJ,
< 3 mm at mid-thigh
< 2 mm at mid-calf

They even suggested that patients with GSV diameter less than those described above should be spared of saphenectomy.

Study by Lane et al suggested that patients with larger truncal vein diameters presented with worse clinical disease severity, as assessed by CEAP and VCSS. But this was not associated with worse quality of life. A diameter >6 mm was associated with a significantly greater quality of life impairment and clinical disease severity. Male patients had higher scoring meaning they suffered worse clinical stage and quality of life

4.9 Image. GSV lumen diameter at SFJ can be helpful in treatment planning.

scores.[4]

(III) PATHOLOGICAL REFLUX (see images 4.10 and 4.11):
Patient position : Evaluated in standing position
Maneuver used : Valsalva's for common femoral and femoral veins; compression for popliteal and calf veins.
Cut off value :[1]
Reflux lasting > 0.5 sec : Superficial veins
　　　　　　　　　　　　　　Deep femoral vein
　　　　　　　　　　　　　　Deep calf veins
Reflux lasting > 1 sec : Femoral and popliteal veins (deep veins)
Reflux lasting > 0.35 sec : Perforators.

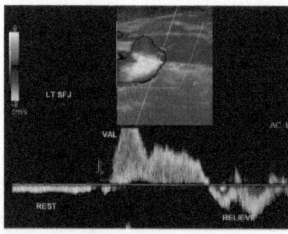

4.10 Image.SFJ REFLUX

Some of the factors assumed to influence duration of reflux are : the vessel diameter, the length of the vessel and number of valves present within the vein. Obviously larger caliber vessel with longer length and less number of valves (as the thigh veins compared to the calf veins), will take longer time to shut off the physiologic reflux.

(IV) COMPRESSIBILITY :
Superficial veins are fairly compressible and that needs to be demonstrated. Thrombosed superficial veins need to be documented, as those might change the approach for venous ablation procedure.

DIAGNOSTIC US FINDINGS – PERFORATORS

(I) LOCATION: Perforator location is important point to document, not only for treatment, but also for follow up purposes. Its communication to deep vein may also be mentioned

(II) REFLUX (see image 4.12):

The commonly used criteria to define reflux in perforators is flow reversal > 0.5 seconds, following manual compression. Abrupt closure of reverse flow is considered competent, regardless of reverse flow duration.[5] As we saw above, the criteria listed was 0.35 seconds. The bottom line though is, with practice you will realize what pathological reflux is, and there may hardly be a difference of 0.35 or 0.5 sec.

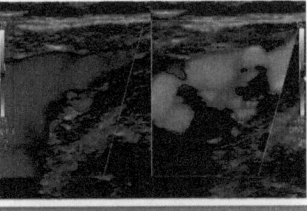

4.11 Image. SFJ reflux on color mode

Manual compression to elicit reflux provides uniformity in evaluating veins with different anatomical orientations.

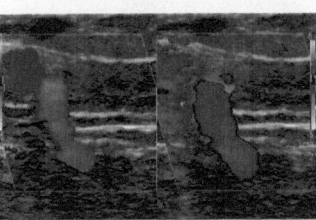

4.12 Image. Incompetent perforator in thigh

(III) DIAMETER: Diameters were measured on B-mode transverse projections at the crossing of the fascia.

Perforator diameter > 3.5 mm no matter where in the lower extremity is highly predictive of pathological reflux.[5]

In this study, the thigh perforating vein diameter > 3.5 mm or larger was predictive of reflux in 92 %, and diameter < 3mm was predicted of reflux in 81%, whereas perforators with diameter < 2.5 mm were all competent.

The calf perforator diameter 3.5 mm or larger was predictive of reflux in 90%, and diameter < 2.2 mm was predictive of lack of reflux in 92% cases.

The suggested calf perforating veins diameter correlation with incompetency: [5]
1.5 mm - normal
2.5 mm – abnormal but competent
3.5 mm – incompetent
4.5 mm – severely incompetent

Increase in the number and diameter of medial calf perforating veins, particularly those permitting bidirectional flow are associated with deteriorating CEAP grade of CVI.[6]

    (IV)   FUNCTIONAL ROLE: of incompetent perforator. For example, the incompetent perforator may be the source of primary incompetence in presence of competent SFJ. Alternatively, the identified incompetent perforator may be the route of drainage for refluxing saphenous vein.

INFORMATION REQUIRED FROM US FOR ENDOVENOUS LASER

Apart from the information obtained from diagnostic ultrasound, namely, presence of reflux, level of reflux, incompetency of perforators, etc., some of the information is specifically relevant to the interventional portion of the exam only. Key points are listed below:

> - GSV diameter < 6 mm : advancing laser / RF fiber could be technically challenging, and may end up extra venous.[2]
> - GSV diameter > 14 mm : Laser / RF may be ineffective; At least external compression and/or

perivenous tumescent anesthesia for good wall apposition required.[2]
- GSV distance from skin (i.e. laser fiber tip from the skin) < 5mm : risk of thermal damage.[2]
- GSV tortuosity : advancing laser / RF fiber is difficult, may have to take multiple accesses and treat segments separately.[2] (see image 4.13 and 4.14).

INCIDENTAL ULTRASOUND FINDINGS

While performing ultrasound for evaluating varicosities, one may encounter incidental findings, which should be documented. These may not be reevaluated with the endovenous laser procedure, but is helpful in follow up. Examples of these may be :

- Arterial aneurysm
- Lymph nodes
- Baker's cyst
- Hematoma
- Soft tissue / osseous mass

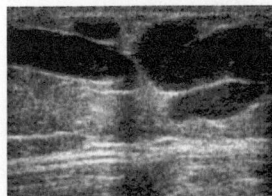

4.13 Image. Tortuous GSV in leg needs attention while planning laser procedure, as the fiber being a linear rigid element may not negotiate through the tortuosity, and may end up in the extraluminal space.

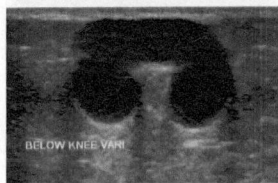

4.14 Image. B mode image of superficial varicosity in leg. Note that this may require sclerosant administration.

OTHER DIAGNOSTIC MODALITIES

Gold standard for localization of reflux – descending venography (invasive).
Gold standard for hemodynamic quantification of reflux – ambulatory venous pressure (invasive).

REFERENCES:

1. Labropoulos N, Tiongson J, Pryor L, et al. Definition of venous reflux in lower-extremity veins. J Vasc Surg 2003;38: 793-8.
2. Cina A[1], Pedicelli A, Di Stasi C, Porcelli A, Fiorentino A, Cina G, Rulli F, Bonomo L.. Color-Doppler sonography in chronic venous insufficiency: what the radiologist should know Curr Probl Diagn Radiol. 2005 Mar-Apr;34(2):51-62.
3. Navarro TP, Delis KT, Ribeiro AP. Clinical and hemodynamic significance of the greater saphenous vein diameter in chronic venous insufficiency. Arch Surg 2002;137:1233-7.
4. Lane, T.R.A. et al. Big Veins, Big Deal - Vein Diameter Affects Disease Severity, not Quality of Life. Journal of Vascular Surgery: Venous and Lymphatic Disorders 2013, 1(1): 101
5. Sandri JL, Barros FS, Pontes S, et al. Diameter-reflux relationship in perforating veins of patients with varicose veins. J Vasc Surg 1999;30:867-75.
6. Stuart WP, Adam DJ, Allan PL, Ruckley CV, Bradbury AW. The relationship between the number, competence, and diameter of medial calf perforating veins and the clinical status in healthy subjects and patients with lower-limb venous disease. J Vasc Surg. 2000 Jul;32(1):138-43.

7. Englehorn CA, Englehorn AL, Cassou MF, Salles-Cunha SX. Patterns of saphenous reflux in women with varicose veins. J Vasc Surg 2005;41: 645-51
8. Gibson, Kathleen D. et al. Endovenous laser treatment of the short saphenous vein: Efficacy and complications. Journal of Vascular Surgery , 2007, 45 (4) : 795 - 803
9. Meissner, Mark H. et al. The hemodynamics and diagnosis of venous disease. J Vasc Surg 2007; 46(6): S4 - S24
10. Cavezzi, N. Labropoulos, H. Partsch, S. Ricci, A. Caggiati, K. Myers, A. Nicolaides, P.C. Smith, Duplex Ultrasound Investigation of the Veins in Chronic Venous Disease of the Lower Limbs— UIP Consensus Document. Part II. Anatomy. Eur J Vasc Endovasc Surg 2006; 31: 288–299
11. Labropoulos N, Leon M, Geroulakos G, Volteas N, Chan P, Nicolaides AN. Venous hemodynamic abnormalities in patients with leg ulceration. Am J Surg. 1995;169(6):572–574.
12. Gloviczki P, Bergan JJ, Rhodes JM, Canton LG, Harmsen S, Ilstrup DM, the North American Study Group Mid-term results of endoscopic perforator vein interruption for chronic venous insufficiency: lessons learned from the North American subfascial endoscopic perforator surgery registry. J Vasc Surg. 1999;29(3):489–502.
13. Perrin M. Surgery for deep venous reflux in the lower limb. J Mal Vasc. 2004 May;29(2):73-87.

Chapter 5

MANAGEMENT TECHNIQUES

1. CONVENTIONAL AND CURRENT TECHNIQUES

The techniques available for management of varicose veins have increased from the traditional surgery to new interventional ones, in the past few years. Various procedures are performed in different institutions and practices with different protocols, and each having valid reasons.

Here, we have briefly listed the procedures pertaining to varicose veins management.

Surgical – stripping and ligation

Up until past few years, this was the only available option for varicose veins. The GSV is flush ligated at the SF junction through a groin incision, and then stripped off using the stripper.

Salient features of this surgery are:
- Improves quality of life.

- Great short-term efficacy.
- Needs to be combined with phlebectomies.
- Does not take into account the perforator incompetence.
- Unacceptable high rate of recurrence. (5 Year recurrence rate approx. 30 % for GSV and 50 % for SSV, presumably due to neovascularization).[3,4]
- Significant postoperative morbidity (bleeding, groin infection, thrombophlebitis, saphenous nerve damage)
- Post-operative scar
- Associated with neurologic damage (40% with GSV stripping, 7 % with SSV stripping).[5,6]
- Requires general/ regional anesthesia

Endovenous laser ablation

Thermal ablation of the vein is performed using laser energy. The fibre is percutaneously introduced in the incompetent superficial vein.
- Improved efficacy compared to surgery
- Reduced postoperative morbidity, including pain and discomfort.
- Early return to routine daily activities and work.
- Can be performed on outpatient basis.
- Can be performed without general/ regional anesthesia (although tumescent anesthesia may be used).
- Ideal for high-risk surgical candidates.
- Laser has higher immediate success rate, is easier, faster and has fewer complications, compared to conventional surgery in treating SSV incompetence.[12]

Endovenous laser ablation has proved to be effective in preventing recurrence of venous ulceration and in treatment of non-healing venous ulcers, much better than compression therapy alone[26]. Effectiveness of ablation techniques for SSV have been successful and durable[27,28,29].

Radiofrequency ablation

- Ablation similar to endovenous laser ablation.
- Conflicting results compared to endovenous laser.
- Better compared to surgery
- Some reports claim less postoperative pain, but similar results to laser.

Sclerotherapy

Sclerosant instilled into the vein under US guidance, which obliterates the vein lumen.
- Due to its liquid form, it mixes with blood and flows along with the blood in venous lumen
- Less invasive of all.
- Short term results comparable.
- Can be used for superficial veins, which due to their morphology, render advancement of laser fiber impossible (eg, very superficial vein or extremely tortuous vein, etc.)
- Can be used for perforator treatment.

Foam sclerotherapy

Involves introduction of foamed sclerosant into the incompetent superficial vein or perforator.

- Similar to the sclerotherapy, but the sclerosant is foamed, which can be prepared using Tessari technique.
- Short term efficacy similar to surgery
- Less post op pain
- Earlier return to normal activities
- Less efficient than other methods (16.3% patent after 1 year)
- Often required multiple sittings.

- Possible complications include: visual disturbance, transient neurological deficits, migraines, deep vein thrombosis (DVT), and superficial phlebitis. Although, in our practice, except for the superficial phlebitis, we did not encounter other complications. We assume that's related to the amount of foam injected and ultrasound guidance, which has been the key.

Sclerosant, as well as sclerosant mixed with air has been in use for several years. There have been several different methods described to prepare foamed sclerosant, some of which include Monfreux method, Cabrera method, Benigni-Sedoun, Garcia mingo, etc.[21] The one which we used at our practice, and which is probably the simplest and easiest is the Tessari's technique, which was described by Lorenzo Tessari in 1999, using two disposable syringes and a three way tap. The foam can be reconstituted several times during the procedure, if the treatment session is prolonged.

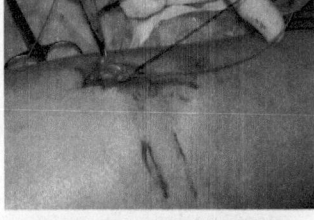

5.1 Image. Perforator ligation surgery

What's the advantage of foam over liquid?

The liquid sclerosant when injected mixes with venous blood and gets diluted. This diluted sclerosant then is available for action on endothelium. The net available concentration of sclerosant is of course highly unpredictable, depending upon its mixing with venous blood.

On the contrary, foam, which is constituted of small bubbles, when injected into the venous blood, displaces blood, and comes into contact with the endothelium. The sclerosant is lined on the surface of the air bubble, and is the same concentration, which was intended for use. Thus, to produce the same effect on endothelium, the net concentration and volume of sclerosant that will be required is low in foamed form as compared to liquid form.

Perforator surgery (image 5.1)

Robert Linton first recommended surgical ligation of the incompetent calf perforators in patients with venous ulcers in 1938. The procedure he described, that consists a long incision along medial leg that provided access to all incompetent veins, is rarely practiced today. Due to frequent associated wound complications, several variations of this procedure were attempted without much ultimate success. Endoscopic visualization however demonstration some promise.

Subfascial endoscopic perforator surgery (SEPS)

Although safety and efficacy has been demonstrated, the indications remain controversial. [11]

The question of perforator surgery gains its importance when there is presence of deep venous reflux, either by itself or in combination with GSV and/or SSV reflux. In these patients treating GSV and/or SSV alone may not be sufficient, and there might be need to deal with the perforators. But there are studies out there, which obviate the need, and recommend dealing with GSV and/or SSV itself that may be sufficient. Either way, we have been dealing with the perforators and in our practice, and we have performed sclerotherapy for these incompetent perforators.

Perforator classification based on the distribution of venous reflux:

Type I :
- supplied by superficial venous reflux
- Deep system normal.

- 80 % of cases refluxing flow from perforator corrected following saphenous surgery alone

Type II :
- No GSV / SSV reflux
- Isolated deep venous reflux.
- Require perforator direct surgical interruption

Type III:
- Superficial venous reflux
- Deep venous reflux
- Saphenous surgery + perforator treatment

Laser Vs RF
Venous clinical severity score (VCSS)
No significant difference is seen in the improvement in mean score following surgery, endovenous laser, radiofrequency ablation or foam sclerotherapy.[2]

Aberdeen Varicose Vein Symptom Severity Score
Even this score had no significant change following the four procedures.

The meta-analysis by van den Bos et al revealed that the minimally invasive techniques were as effective as surgery, and endovenous ablation is significantly more effective than RF ablation in obliterating the insufficient veins.[7]

There have been other studies which reported that endovenous laser was superior to RF ablation.[8] Out there are also studies which report that laser and RF ablation were equally effective.[9]

And needless to say, you will find studies demonstrating superiority of RF ablation over endovenous laser.[10]

Microphlebectomy

Phlebectomy refers to surgical vein removal that requires a large incision on an already diseased skin and subcutaneous tissue, rendering its healing a prolonged process. Microphlebectomy has smaller incisions through which the hooked devices are advanced to remove abnormal vein. This is associated with less blood loss, post-operative pain and scarring, and do not require sutures. Moreover, the abnormal vein is removed forever.

2. OTHER NEWER TECHNIQUES

The ablation techniques have proven to be very effective as minimally invasive procedures. More new techniques are directed towards making procedures less painful and tolerable but need to prove their efficacy comparable to ablation techniques. World over different methods have been and are being tried and reported.

Foam washout sclerotherapy

K.Fattahi[13] reported this foam washout sclerotherapy. The suggested mechanism of action of sclerosant is its contact with endothelium. It is believed that contact of sclerosant with the endothelium for a few seconds is sufficient to cause damage. Thereafter, presence of sclerosant in the vein and in the systemic circulation is not required, which is believed to reduce incidence of complications. We personally have not worked with this technique, and since we personally were comfortable with foam sclerosant (not the foam washout), we may not be able to comment on this. Theoretically, though this has a logical reason, its long-term results and efficacy would be interesting to know. The technique is to secure separate venous access for injecting and aspirating the foam into and from the vein being treated. On one end the foamed sclerosant is injected, and this then is aspirated from the other venous access, providing just few seconds for the sclerosant to be in contact with the endothelium.

MOCA[23]

Mechanico-chemical ablation (MOCA) is a new technique involving mechanical damage to venous endothelium and infusion of sclerosant in liquid form. The damage is caused by a catheter which is introduced in a similar fashion as the ablation laser / RF fibers. The catheter is positioned peripheral to SFJ as in the ablation techniques. The activated catheter has rotating tip, and disperses liquid sclerosant to the venous wall being damaged simultaneously.

- No heating of vein is involved, so no tumescent anesthesia is required
- Less postoperative pain compared to RF/ laser ablation.
- Short term follow up results comparable to ablation techniques.
- Long-term results and efficacy are yet awaited.
- Potential for nerve damage is minimized, as thermal energy is not involved.

A multicenter randomized control trial; MESSI (Mechanochemical Endovenous ablation versus radiofrequency ablation in the treatment of primary Small Saphenous vein Insufficiency) will reveal the results of MOCA compared to RF ablation. The trial planned to enroll patients through 3rd quarter of 2015. Subsequently the 1-year follow up and thereafter results could be available.

COMBINED LASER ABLATION AND GSV LIGATION

A variation of endovenous laser ablation has been surgical ligation of GSV 1-2 cm peripheral to the SFJ. Additionally, venous tributaries in vicinity of the SFJ are also ligated. It has been proposed that this may have better hemodynamic effects, and is used to prevent recanalization and deep venous thrombosis related to femoral vein ablation.[15,16]

STEAM GSV ABLATION[22]

This is another endovascular technique to cause GSV ablation, but using steam vein sclerosis system. This again is related to delivery of thermal energy, which induces endothelial damage. The technique is more or less similar to the endovenous laser procedure with some instrumentation differences.

VALVULOPLASTY

Reconstruction of venous valve by creating valve cusps via dissection into the thickened venous wall was reported by Maleti and Lugli[19,20]. The procedure has been performed in patients with deep venous insufficiency, either of post-thrombotic origin or congenital valve agenesis. Short and mid-term efficacies have been reported but long-term results are awaited. It appears to be effective in restoring femoral competence.

There are other methods and techniques described as well with varying results and published in various journals worldwide. Some of these techniques include direct valvuloplasty, femoral vein transposition, venous segment transplantation, cryopreserved vein valve, inverted saphenous vein segment, etc. The long-term effects of modified neovalve reconstruction procedures are yet to be validated.

MANAGEMENT OF ULCER

Whatever technique we use for managing the superficial venous reflux, the presence of active/ recurrent ulcer also needs management.

Note: Presence of active venous ulcer does not preclude from performing the laser ablation procedure. Presence of active cellulitis though may require a course of antibiotic. Even presence of purulent exudate is not a contraindication for laser procedure.

For ulcer management, key component of care is cleanliness and sterility. The area needs to be kept clean by the patient, and needs regular non-adhesive absorbent sterile dressing. Therefore, self-care of ulcer is of utmost importance.

The addition of endovenous laser ablation for refluxing GSV fastens the process of ulcer healing and preventing recurrence. The presence of uncorrected deep venous reflux has no effect on initial healing time[17]. There is no significant difference in time to heal or the long-term ulcer healing between patients who did or did not use compression stocking following interventional procedure. In fact, compression stocking may be unnecessary to fasten initial ulcer healing or prevent late recurrences, following interventional procedure.[17,18] However, the compression stockings do have a role in controlling limb swelling and symptoms related to it. There is no need to apply topical antibiotics or chemicals, particularly to the ulcers defined as small in size. Large size ulcers may require skin graft placement adjunctive to the laser ablation procedure.

Ulcer healing for small ulcers (<500mm^2 or approx. 1 inch size) is faster compared to the large size ulcers (≥500 mm^2). More than 80% of small ulcers heal by 14 weeks following the laser procedure.

Chronic non-healing ulcers may require a combination of approach, ranging from conservative to more aggressive plastic surgery approach, while addressing the underlying etiology of venous reflux[24,25].

REFERENCES:

1. Stuart WP, Adam DJ, Allan PL, Ruckley CV, Bradbury AW.Saphenous surgery does not correct perforator incompetencein the presence of deep venous reflux. J Vasc Surg 1998;28:834-8.
2. L. H. Rasmussen, M. Lawaetz, L. Bjoern, B. Vennits, A. Blemings and B. Eklof. Randomized clinical trial comparing endovenous laser ablation, radiofrequency ablation, foam sclerotherapy and surgical stripping for great saphenous varicose veins.British Journal of Surgery 2011; 98: 1079–1087
3. Hartmann K, Klode J, Pfister R, Toussaint M, Weingart I, Waldermann F, et al. Recurrent varicose veins: sonography-based re-examination of 210 patients 14 years after ligation and saphenous vein stripping. Vasa 2006;35:21-6.
4. Darke SG. The morphology of recurrent varicose veins. Eur J Vasc Surg 1992;6:512-7.
5. Morrison C, Dalsing MC. Signs and symptoms of saphenous nerve injury after greater saphenous vein stripping: prevalence, severity,and relevance for modern practice. J Vasc Surg 2003;38:886-90.
6. Holmes JB, Skajaa K, Holme K. Incidence of lesions of the saphenous nerve after partial or complete stripping of the long saphenous vein. Acta Chir Scand 1990;156:145-8.
7. van den Bos, Renate et al. Endovenous therapies of lower extremity varicosities: A meta-analysis. Journal of Vascular Surgery , 2009; 49 (1) : 230 - 239
8. Almeida JI, Raines JK. Radiofrequency ablation and laser ablation in the treatment of varicose veins. Ann Vasc Surg 2006;20547–52.
9. Puggioni A, Kalra M, Carmo M, Mozes G, Gloviczki P. Endovenous laser therapy and radiofrequency ablation of the great saphenous

vein: analysis of early efficacy and complications. J Vasc Surg 2005;42:488-93.
10. Shepherd AC, Gohel MS, Brown LC, Metcalfe MJ, Hamish M, Davies AH. Randomized clinical trial of VNUS ClosureFAST radiofrequency ablation versus laser for varicose veins. Br J Surg 2010; **97**: 810–818.
11. Coleridge Smith P. Calf perforating veins—Time for an objective appraisal? Phlebology 1996;11:135-6.
12. Roopram, Avinash D. et al. Endovenous laser ablation versus conventional surgery in the treatment of small saphenous vein incompetence. J Vasc Surg: Venous and Lym Dis 2013;1:357-63
13. K.Fattahi. Foam Washout Sclerotherapy: A New Technique Geared Toward Reducing Short- and Long-term Complications of Regular Foam Sclerotherapy and Comparison with Existing Foam Sclerotherapy Method. JOURNAL OF VASCULAR SURGERY: VENOUS AND LYMPHATIC DISORDERS; 2013;1(1): 111
14. van Eekeren, Ramon R.J.P. et al. Mechanochemical endovenous ablation for the treatment of great saphenous vein insufficiency.J Vasc Surg: Venous and Lym Dis. 2014;2:282-8
15. Zhu HP, Zhou YL, Zhang X, Yan JL, Xu ZY, Wang H, et al. Combined endovenous laser therapy and pinhole high ligation in the treatment of symptomatic great saphenous varicose veins. Ann Vasc Surg 2014;28:301-5.
16. Park Y, Young-Wook Kim, Yang-Jin Park, et al.Postoperative hemodynamic changes after endovenous laser ablation and phlebectomy in varicose vein surgery.(J Vasc Surg: Venous and Lym Dis 2015;3:54-7.)
17. Raju, Seshadri et al. Endovenous management of venous leg ulcers .J Vasc Surg: Venous and Lym Dis 2013;1:165-73
18. Scriven JM, Hartshorne T, Thrush AJ, Bell PR, Naylor AR, London NJ. Role of saphenous vein

surgery in the treatment of venous ulceration. Br J Surg 1998;85:781-4.
19. Maleti O, Lugli M. Neovalve construction in postthrombotic syndrome.J Vasc Surg 2006;43:794-9.
20. Lugli M, Guerzoni S, Garofalo M, Smedile G, Maleti O. Neovalve construction in deep venous incompetence. J Vasc Surg 2009;49: 156-62; 62 e1-2; discussion: 162.
21. Frullini A, Cavezzi A. Sclerosing foam in the treatment of varicose veins and telangiectases: history and analysis of safety and complications. Dermatol Surg. 2002 Jan;28(1):11-5.
22. Mlosek RK[1], Woźniak W, Gruszecki L, Stapa RZ.The use of a novel method of endovenous steam ablation in treatment of great saphenous vein insufficiency: own experiences. Phlebology. 2014 Feb;29(1):58-65.
23. Boersma D, van Eekeren RR, Kelder HJ, et al. Mechanochemical endovenous ablation versus radiofrequency ablation in the treatment of primary small saphenous vein insufficiency (MESSI trial): study protocol for a randomized controlled trial. Trials. 2014;15:421. doi:10.1186/1745-6215-15-421.
24. Alamelu V. Is chronic venous ulcer curable? A sample survey of a plastic surgeon. Indian Journal of Plastic Surgery : Official Publication of the Association of Plastic Surgeons of India. 2011;44(1):104-109. doi:10.4103/0970-0358.81457.
25. Kumins NH, Weinzweig N, Schuler JJ. Free tissue transfer provides durable treatment for large nonhealing venous ulcers. J Vasc Surg 2000;32:848-54.
26. Marston WA. Efficacy of endovenous ablation of the saphenous veins for prevention and healing of venous ulcers. J Vasc Surg: Venous and LymDis 2015;3:113-6.
27. Gibson KD, Ferris BL, Polissar N,Neradilek B, Pepper D. Endovenous laser treatment of the

short saphenous vein: efficacy and complications. J Vasc Surg 2007; 45:795–801.
28. Proebstle TM, Gul D, Kargl A, Knop J. Endovenous Laser treatment of the lesser saphenous vein with a 940-nm diode laser: early results. Dermatol Surg 2003;29:357-61.
29. Ravi R, Rodriguez-Lopez JA, Traylor EA, Barrett DA, Ramaiah V, Diethrich EB. Endovenous ablation of incompetent saphenous veins: a large single-center experience. J Endovasc Ther 2006;13:244-8.

Chapter 6

PATIENT SELECTION FOR ENDOVENOUS LASER

Patient selection becomes pretty much simpler if we define patients that may not be ideal candidates for the endovenous laser procedure, since that list is much shorter compared to the list of those in whom the procedure is indicated.

Absolute contraindications

Conditions that precluded us from treating varicose veins using with endovenous laser were:
1. Acute deep vein thrombosis.
2. Recently documented partially recanalized deep vein thrombosis.
3. Certain etiologies of varicose veins, which need to be managed first, for example, an abdominal and/or pelvic mass compressing the venous outflow from pelvis thereby mechanically impeding venous return from lower extremities.

Relative contraindications

1. Ongoing risk for thrombosis, severe uncorrectable coagulopathy and liver dysfunction: Benefit versus risk needs to be assessed in these scenarios. The risk may be reduced with prophylactic anticoagulants. A recent or active venous thromboembolism also needs consideration.
2. Pregnant patients – because of concern for anesthetic use and unknown impact of heated blood that fetus may be exposed to. Additionally, post-partum evaluation of lower extremity veins would provide a more accurate assessment of underlying reflux, once the pelvic compression of iliac veins and IVC is relieved.
3. Breast-feeding patients.
4. Allergy to local anesthetics – Alternatives include cold saline and vocal anesthesia.
5. Developmental anomalies, for example, Klippel-Trenaunay Syndrome (KTS): A thorough anatomical review of venous map needs to be performed to confirm adequate deep venous return in the event that the abnormal superficial channels are ablated.
6. Isolated incompetent deep veins: Aggressive management may be considered if conservative management has failed, and patient's symptoms are refractory, particularly chronic non-healing and/or recurrent ulcer[1,2]. There have been reports of improved deep venous reflux following stripping of a refluxing GSV. However, incomplete stripping may lead to development of new deep venous reflux in the femoral and popliteal veins[3].
7. Allergy to polidocanol or sodium tetradecyl sulfate: in patients being planned for sclerotherapy, either as an individual procedure or in combination with other procedures.
8. Immobility after the procedure: This may hamper the expected response from the procedure, and may additionally pose the risk for deep vein thrombosis. A sequential compression device or pneumatic compression device could be used in these cases.
9. Ongoing systemic infection.
10. Poor general health.

Conditions not excluded from treatment:

1. Concomitant perforator incompetence with GSV incompetence.
2. Concomitant SSV incompetence with GSV incompetence.
3. Prior history of GSV ablation and/or surgical treatment.

Common concerns for clinicians

Question: Is endovenous laser safe in patients on warfarin, Coumadin or antiplatelet medications?
Answer: It is safe with the international normalized ratio between 2 and 3. There is no need to interrupt these medications, as there is no adverse effect of anticoagulation or antiplatelet therapy on closure rates of the vein, and there is no major bleeding complication. However, each case needs to be assessed individually and other risk factors and health conditions still need to be considered.

Question: The tortuous abnormal vein is thrombosed, or has synechiae within it. Would it be feasible to treat this vein with laser?
Answer: Yes, it's possible. Multiple venous accesses may be required unless the entire course of vein is completely thrombosed, in which case the reflux is by default absent.

Question: Is there a benefit of treating enlarged but competent superficial veins?
Answer: No, that's not been proven, and should not be performed.

REFERENCES:

1. Sales CM, Bilof ML, Petrillo KA, Luka NL. Correction of lower extremity deep venous incompetence by ablation of superficial venous reflux. Ann Vasc Surg

1996; 10:186.
2. Puggioni A, Lurie F, Kistner RL, Eklof B. How often is deep venous reflux eliminated after saphenous vein ablation? J Vasc Surg 2003; 38:517.
3. MacKenzie RK, Allan L, Ruckley CV, et al. Effect of long saphenous vein stripping on deep venous reflux. Eur J Vasc Endovasc Surg. 2004;28:104-7.
4. Effect of anticoagulation on endothermal ablation of the great saphenous vein. Sharifi, Mohsen et al. Journal of Vascular Surgery, Volume 53, Issue 1, 147 – 149

Chapter 7

CONCEPT OF LASER APPLICATION IN VARICOSE VEINS TREATMENT

LASER is the acronym for "Light Amplification by Stimulated Emission of Radiation". It's an optical amplification that is based on stimulated emission of electromagnetic radiation. This creates a high-energy coherent light that is monochromatic (one wavelength). Laser has several applications in diverse fields, and medical field is one of them.

Mechanisms of Action and Debate on Different Laser Wavelengths

Laser has established itself as a successful mode of treatment of varicose veins. The exact mechanism, or to say in other words, what happens at the instance when laser is emitted at the fiber tip within the lumen is not entirely clear. But, ultrasound provides a means to visualize the manifestation and unfolding of events in the vein. The intense temperature at fiber tip (approximately 800 degrees centigrade) drops down to 90 degrees, at a distance of 4 mm from the fiber. From the in vitro experiments, it is believed to result from energy absorption by de-oxyhemoglobin of venous blood[1]. This intense energy absorption by venous blood causes boiling and bubbles formation[2].

Histologically, the endothelium, intimal layer and media are damaged following laser ablation. The adventitia is affected in some cases[3]. However, the peak temperature adjoining the vein, from studies on pigs, usually did not exceed 50 degrees[4]. The penetration of laser beam into blood is only a few mm, for example, 0.3 mm in a 940 nm laser[1]. This low penetration could explain the focal venous wall perforation in the vicinity of firing laser fiber tip, but not a widespread venous wall injury. Therefore, it was proposed in different studies that bubble formation was related to extensive thermal vein wall injury[2,5].

Whatever their origin, the bubbles remain loco-regional and have not shown to pose risk for pulmonary embolism. They are a short-lived phenomenon that lasts only until the fiber is firing.

Basic components of any laser system include an energy supply, a lasing medium (semiconductors in case of diode lasers), optical cavity and optical deliver system. Each laser bare fiber has a silica core, and cladding (silica or hard plastic). A plastic covering encases the fiber, which terminates 4-8 mm proximal to distal end of emitting tip[6].

Proebstle et al used 940 nm Diode laser to study the effects on venous wall. They delivered the laser energy in a pulsed fashion into the GSV, with 1 second on and 2 second off period. During the 1 sec on period, they delivered the laser energy. During the 2 second off period, they retracted the laser fiber by 5-7mm. When they studied the histopathology of the treated GSV, it shows two different patterns. At the site of direct laser action was perforating and non-perforating vaporization of venous wall, carbonization of adjacent tissue margins explosion like intimal tear. In the 5-7 mm intervening segments between the direct impacts of laser fiber, heat injury was noted. Additionally, they performed in vitro evaluation of laser-induced effect on blood, which revealed steam bubble formation during the delivery of laser energy, which collapses on discontinuing laser energy.

The widespread injury to the venous wall is not simply explained by focal laser energy delivery by fiber tip or by contact with venous wall. There has to be something else adding to the job.

Vuylsteke et al described in their article in 2012, that the physical properties of water, the bubble in Proebstle et al study constituted only 1.6% of the total energy delivered[7]. Besides, the boiling zone is within the lumen, and the vapors collapse when they reach a cooler area. The bubbles have a little impact on the venous wall. Additionally, the histopathological samples were from the vein that was treated immediately prior to obtaining sections.

But before we review other possible mechanisms, lets mention that the direct contact has its own role, and the destruction of venous wall and its impact on perivenous structures extend beyond the 1 week duration, and is believed to be the cause of post-operative pain, inflammation and ecchymosis.

Laser light can be absorbed, scattered or reflected, the latter though is very minimal in infrared spectrum. Absorption is based on light absorbing elements in biological tissues called the chromophores (e.g., hemoglobin, water, melanin, etc.), which have different absorption coefficients. Since the laser is monochromatic light, chromophores can be selectively targeted. The 810, 940, and 980 nm lasers are absorbed by deoxygenated hemoglobin. The 980 nm laser are also absorbed by intracellular water, as are the laser of wavelengths higher than 980 nm.

Optical extinction, which is based on absorption and scattering coefficient, is higher at higher wavelengths, such as 1470 nm compared to 810 nm. The optical extinction for blood and vessel wall is similar for most of the wavelengths. Therefore, Vuylsteke et al mentioned that the classification based on blood-absorbed and water-absorbed laser wavelengths is inappropriate[7]. There are two more points that are reinforced by this understanding. The optical extinction being similar for blood and water, it's important to empty intraluminal blood so that water (and therefore the venous wall) is preferred by laser energy. Else, the absorption by blood leads to thrombotic occlusion and possible recanalization later. Since the optical extinction with higher wavelengths is higher, this could lead to more venous wall and/or perivenous destruction for the same amount of energy delivered. Therefore, when using lasers of higher wavelengths, less of energy is required to produce the same effect. It should be remembered though; the only exception to above discussion is 810 nm lasers, which has higher optical extinction for vessel wall over blood.

The heat pipe mechanism suggests that vein itself acts as heat pipe when a coagulum composed of steam bubbles at the fiber tip acts as mode of heat conduction at constant temperature from laser tip to the venous wall. Inflammatory markers are seen in perivenous space in weeks following the laser delivery, which subsequently leads to fibrous scar formation over time.

So, that's clear, higher the intraluminal blood volume, lesser will be the wall destruction, which otherwise is the goal of this treatment. Empty your veins prior to laser delivery. This can be augmented by perivenous tumescent local anesthesia infiltration, and/or by Trendelenburg position also.

Massaki et al discussed the same concepts in 2013, although they talked about hemoglobin and myoglobin in vein wall as main chromophores at low end of wavelength spectrum, and water in the venous wall as the main chromophores at the higher wavelength spectrum[8].

The debate continued in 2014 with publication from Poluektova et al, who concluded that, the presumed advantage of wavelengths targeting water rather than hemoglobin is flawed[9].

Pulse versus Continuous Mode

PULSE MODE

The laser energy in this mode is turned on for certain duration, and then turned off. During the turn off time, the laser fiber can be withdrawn by certain distance, following which the laser can be turned on again, and so forth. Consider an example where a laser is set to fire for 1 second, and then off for 1 second. During the off time, fiber is withdrawn at distance felt to be appropriate (say for example 2mm). The laser fiber fires again for a period of 1 second during which time the fiber is kept stationary. Now, if the fiber is moved by 2mm during the off period, it takes 5 such off periods of 1 sec to get the fiber across by 1 cm. That means 5 periods of laser firings, each of 1 second would be delivered across that 1 cm. Since, Joules = Watts x second, the Joules delivered in that 1 cm of vein segment can be calculated by Watts settings of laser machine x 5 seconds.

In short, the above example can be deduced as:

J = W x sec

If the W was 10 W, and we know that 5 seconds of laser firing were required to cover 1 cm of vein segment, then

J = 10 W x 5 sec = 50 Joules.

This, in effect, is the Linear Endovenous Energy Density LEED in this case.

CONTINOUS MODE

During this mode, the laser fiber-sheath complex is pulled back at a relatively constant speed. The LEED here can be calculated by Watts X inverse of pull back speed.

i.e. W X sec/cm

In other words, using higher wattage allows increasing the pullback speed. The slow pull back speed though is of concern in low wavelength lasers (810 nm) which potential can be the vein perforating wavelength and could result in perivenous laser energy delivery[10].

Laser Energy Related Terminologies

FLUENCE

Fluence (J/cm^2) is the single most important parameter that quantifies delivered energy. But since the venous wall surface area (cm^2) is a difficult measurement, LEED (in J/cm) is used as surrogate marker of fluence[15].

LEED

Amongst the various calculations and figures, a threshold of 20 J/ cm^2 was suggested for endovenous laser ablation of GSV, which translates to 6.3 J/cm for each mm of vein diameter[11]. So, if you have a 10 mm vein diameter, then delivering 63 J/cm should be the desired LEED. Increasing the dose of laser energy has shown 100% immediate success rate and significant reduction in recanalization in 12-month follow up[11]. Some have increased the LEED to 95 J/cm with success, although using the tumescent anesthesia[12].

There are other studies, which have worked on energy dosing, and continuous mode and have emphasized the importance to continuous wave over pulse wave delivery, since the former cauterizes the intermittent vein instead of the intermittent vein segments[14].

The debate is ongoing, but for satisfaction of the reader, reference to mathematical model is recommended, which was published in 2006, and reported that both pulse and continuous mode of laser delivery are efficient. Continuous mode may be a faster technique and damages the vein along entire length, but pulse mode is equally successful and the interesting observation was less energy required by pulse mode than continuous mode[16]. This mathematical model suggested that 65 and 100 J/cm was needed for varicose veins of 3 and 5 mm respectively, for irreversible intimal destruction.

WATTAGE

Administering high wattage for a short time has a vaporizing effect and low wattage for longer time has a coagulating effect[3]. Using low wattage can be as effective, and with low side effects, as shown on the study involving 980 nm[13]. Our experience has been the same with 980 nm.

REFERENCES:

1. A. Roggan, M. Friebel, K. Dörschel, A. Hahn, G.J. Mueller. Optical properties of circulating human blood in the wavelength range 400–2500 nm. J Biomed Opt, 4 (1999), pp. 36–46
2. T.M. Proebstle, H.A. Lehr, A. Kargl, C. Espinola-Klein, W. Rother, S. Bethge, et al. Endovenous treatment of the greater saphenous vein with a 940-nm diode laser: thrombotic occlusion after endoluminal thermal damage by laser-generated steam bubbles. J Vasc Surg, 35 (2002), pp. 729–736
3. L. Corcos, S. Dini, D. De Anna, O. Marangoni, E. Ferlaino, T. Procacci, et al. The immediate effects of endovenous diode 808-nm laser in the greater saphenous vein: morphologic study and clinical implications. J Vasc Surg, 41 (2005), pp. 1018–1024
4. S.E. Zimmet, R.J. Min. Temperature changes in perivenous tissue during endovenous laser treatment in a swine model. J Vasc Interv Radiol, 14 (2003), pp. 911–915
5. Sadick NS, Prieto VG, Shea CR, et al. Clinical and pathophysiologic correlates of 1064-nm Nd.YAG laser treatment of reticular veins and venulectasias. Arch Dermatol 2001;137:613-7.
6. Vuylsteke et al. Endovenous Laser Ablation: A Review of Mechanisms of Action. Ann Vasc Surg 2012; 26: 424–433
7. Vuylsteke et al. Endovenous Laser Ablation: A Review of Mechanisms of Action. Ann Vasc Surg 2012; 26: 424–433
8. Massaki A et al. Endoluminal Laser Delivery Mode and Wavelength Effects on Varicose Veins in an Ex Vivo Model; Lasers in Surgery and Medicine 45:123–129 (2013)
9. Poluektova et al. Some controversies in endovenous laser ablation of varicose veins addressed by optical-

thermal mathematical modeling. Lasers Med Sci. 2014 Mar;29(2):441-52.
10. Weiss RA. Comparison of endovenous radiofrequency versus 810 nm diode laser occlusion of large veins in an animal model. Dermatol Surg 2002;28:56-61.
11. Proebstle TM, Moehler T, Herdemann S. Reduced recanalization rates of the great saphenous vein after endovenous laser treatment with increased energy dosing: definition of a threshold for the endovenous fluence equivalent. J Vasc Surg. 2006; 44: 834–9
12. Paul E. Timperman, Prospective Evaluation of Higher Energy Great Saphenous Vein Endovenous Laser Treatment, Journal of Vascular and Interventional Radiology, Volume 16, Issue 6, June 2005, Pages 791-794
13. H.S. Kim, I.J. Nwankwo, K. Hong, P.S.J. McElgunn. Lower energy endovenous laser ablation of the great saphenous vein with 980 nm diode laser in continuous mode. Cardiovasc Intervent Radiol, 29 (2006), pp. 64–69
14. Satokawa H, Yokoyama H, Wakamatsu H, Igarashi T. Comparison of Endovenous Laser Treatment for Varicose Veins with High Ligation Using Pulse Mode and without High Ligation Using Continuous Mode and Lower Energy. *Annals of Vascular Diseases*. 2010;3(1):46-51. doi:10.3400/avd.AVDoa09008.
15. R.R. van den Bos, M.A. Kockaert, H.A.M. Neumann, T. Nijsten, Technical Review of Endovenous Laser Therapy for Varicose Veins, European Journal of Vascular and Endovascular Surgery, Volume 35, Issue 1, January 2008, Pages 88-95
16. S.R. Mordon, B. Wassmer, J. Zemmouri. Mathematical modeling of endovenous laser treatment (ELT). Biomed Eng Online, 5 (2006), p. 26

Chapter 8

PRE-OPERATIVE WORK UP PRIOR TO ENDOVENOUS LASER

1. Informed consent: Besides being a mandatory requirement, discussing the procedure details, its expected outcomes, possible complications and post procedure care, with the patient, and in appropriate clinical situations with family as well, provides excellent patient outcomes, and goes a long way to build one's own esteemed practice.

2. Choice of Anesthesia: The procedure may be performed under local anesthesia, conscious sedation, spinal anesthesia, general anesthesia and sometimes combination of those. The choice is based on a patient's body habitus, risk factors, venous anatomy, the disease extent, and post-procedural travel plans. The procedure typically is designed to be an outpatient procedure and can be performed under local and/or tumescent anesthesia. In our practice, the choice of anesthesia we have

used was predominantly based on patient's disease extent, since the procedure may involve a combination of endovenous laser and sclerosant injection. A representative example of this could be a clinical situation wherein a patient has bilateral large venous ulcers with incompetent perforators adjoining the ulcers. The incompetent perforators may have to be approached closer to the ulcer margins, which may be pain provoking, uncomfortable to patient, as well as the operator. The successful outcome may then be affected if treatment is suboptimal. This patient may require spinal anesthesia.

3. Preoperative lab work: The blood work which may not be typically must-be-done in all patients, but is recommended, especially if they have not had those in past one month. The test results which operator may want to have include (but not limited to): CBC, Coagulation profile (INR, PT/PTT, platelet count), HIV, HbsAg, Blood glucose (fasting/random).

4. Preoperative anesthesia work up: If patient is undergoing spinal or general anesthesia, he/she needs to be appropriately evaluated by an anesthesiologist to assess their fitness for anesthesia. This work up should preferably be done by the anesthesiologist being involved in the procedure not only due to obvious reasons, but establish a professional rapport with the patient.

5. Formulating plan for hospital stay: Patients have their personal preferences in terms of hospital stay. The procedure, as mentioned before, may be an outpatient procedure, and if there is a facility for post procedure care for couple of hours at the site where procedure is performed, the patient may be observed in that post procedure bay/area. However, certain situations require hospital stay, for example, insurance requirements, patient's comorbid conditions, patients postoperative complains, when

procedure is performed on an out of town patient in later part of the day, etc.

6. Financial clarity: The laser machine, laser fiber, the required set up and equipment's have sizeable costs. It is advised that the mode of payment, the amount, and covered facilities included in that amount, be decided with patient beforehand. If it's insurance company, pre-authorization can be obtained by prescribed means. But the terms of insurance policies should be discussed with patient and insurance company, as this is out of scope of this book. However, to our best knowledge, the only emergency pertaining to treatment of varicose veins, wherein you would prefer the procedure over discussing insurance and/or payment issues, is acute profusely bleeding varicosities. Management of bleeding supersedes the elective choice of procedure.

7. PHOTOS: Obtaining initial photograph of affected extremities helps by having a baseline image. Comparing the subsequent photographs in follow up provides an assessment of morphologic change in disease. The symptomatic relief or worsening is of course what clinician pays attention to, but it can be subjective. Ulcers are a good example since they can be assessed for healing components and size. Other parameters that can be evaluated are extremity discoloration, visible tortuous veins, leg swelling, etc.

8. CLINICAL SCORING / EVALUATION: The simplest way to evaluate clinical score is to ask a patient to describe the intensity rate or provide a score to their clinical complains, on a scale of 1-10, or 1-5, whichever is suitable to the clinician, as long as the scale used is consistent. This can provide a patient's assessment, which then can be compared on the follow up imaging. The "C" Clinical component of CEAP classification is a valuable tool that described

the clinical picture of the disease in a particular patient. The Venous clinical severity score (VCSS) provides a format that can allow for validated clinical assessment.

9. **EXPLAINING EXPECTED CLINICAL OUTCOMES:** Needless to say, clinicians do that in their routine practice. For the outcomes related to endovenous laser procedure, it helps in short and long run, when a patient's family members know what can be expected following the procedure. For example, the tightness along the course of treated vein may be an expected feeling, and need not be taken as an alarming sign. Though, they need to know when these presentations need to be considered as alarming. This may alleviate a patient's and his/her family member's anxiety and apprehension related to post-procedure outcomes, and serve as a boon to treating clinician (and in some cases referring clinician as well).

The most common question, which should be answered even before asked, is: Will my visible veins disappear following the procedure? And a common expectation is that they vanish immediately or within few days. This should be appropriately and honestly answered and explained that the dilated tortuous veins may take few days to few weeks to shrink in size but some may not reveal a significant change in the appearance. These however can be evaluated on follow up exams.

Depending upon a patient's baseline clinical condition, and the response of individual disease condition to the initial treatment, there may be requirement for subsequent procedure as an adjunct or as a part of recurrence. This needs to be explained to the patient. A strategy that we found helpful in our practice is the explanation of underlying pathophysiology, the natural progression of disease, mechanisms responsible for residual versus recurrence, and incidences of recurrence, to patients prior to treatment.

10. PROVIDING CHARTS AND DIAGRAMS: Visual explanations are east to understand and last longer in memory than words. In our practice, we had models, charts and diagrams of legs, which we used to explain patients their venous anatomy, abnormality and ultrasound findings. It is critically important for them to understand various possible venous reflux mechanisms that can potentially be the cause of residual or recurrent disease, and why it's important to deal with all of them.

11. EXPLAINING WARNING SIGNS: Though EVLT is usually a daycare procedure and the patient is back on his feet, explaining warning signs of DVT, such as infection in an preexisting ulcer, any respiratory difficulty, any bleeding from orifices, swelling of legs, fever, thrombophlebitis in the vein, and elastic allergies from stockings, is imperative.

12. Calf exercises: Besides explaining the treatment, it's prudent to recommend the calf exercises as is relevant to each individual case. Since people tend to take this as a broad vague term, and an individual's perception may vary, the best outcomes may be expected if a clinician can help patient build an initial program, so that the exercises can be incorporated in post-procedure daily routine.

13. Compression stockings: Emphasize the importance of wearing compression stockings and how it affects the disease process. Besides this, patients need to be educated about the appropriate technique to put on the stockings, and what time duration of the day they need to wear. Simply putting them on when you rest at night in reclining position is not going to be a wise choice.

14. Build a follow up schedule: This is quite variable for each patient, not only due to the disease factor, but also due to distances these patients may have to travel for follow up visits, and insurance reimbursement factors. Having said that, it is exceedingly efficient to manage chronic venous insufficiency when you set up follow up schedules for your patient's, which can be appropriately modified based on clinical improvement or worsening.

15. Drive back home: It is advisable to have somebody with the patient on the procedure day, who can provide a drive back home. Although we encourage ambulation following the procedure, and immediate return to routine activities, patient may hesitate to drive back on their own.

Chapter 9

ENDOVENOUS LASER TECHNIQUE

Venous mapping and marking (see table 9.1, and images 9.2 and 9.3)

The GSV course may be mapped using ultrasound, and marked on skin using marker pen. This can be done prior to getting patient on procedure table or when patient is taken on the procedure table itself, prior to sterile prepping.

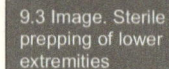
9.3 Image. Sterile prepping of lower extremities

It should be noted though that the absence of deep venous thrombosis needs to be ascertained prior to setting the patient up for procedure, since the whole exercise would be futile if a chronic occlusive / nearly occlusive

9.2 Image. Pre-procedure mapping of GSV

(or possibly an acute DVT) is found out on the procedure table.

> **Chart 9.1. Keypoints to remember**
>
> <u>Venous mapping and marking</u>
>
> - Skin marking
> - Rule out DVT
> - Target vein tortuosity rendering guidewire passage difficult
> - Aneurysmal vein segment
> - Proximity of target vein to the nerve
> - Post-thrombotic synechiae
> - Proximity of target vein to skin

The significance of an initial diagnostic ultrasound scanning (not to be confused with mapping) is in identifying highest and lowest level of reflux in GSV, both of which serve as markers for craniocaudal geographic extent of laser ablation of the vein. Additionally, the presence and location of perforators is identified, a key piece of information required to plan the type of management technique(s). The possibility of adjuvant sclerotherapy can then be discussed with patient beforehand accordingly.

For most part, it's the high frequency linear transducer is what we have been using for superficial venous system.

In our practice, we usually start mapping from sapheno-femoral junction (SFJ). Having ascertained patency and compressibility of common femoral vein at groin, level of SFJ is marked. The GSV is then traced down into the thigh, along medial aspect of knee and leg down to the ankle. Scanning initially in a transverse plane helps excluding the prominent tributaries of GSV that may simulate the GSV itself. In some cases, the GSV may be prominent in thigh proximally, beyond the entry site of tributary draining into it, but may have normal caliber distally.

The highest point of reflux in GSV is marked. This can be taken as the starting point of laser treatment (not the skin entry site). However, skin entry point may be marked inferior to this level, depending upon the lowest point of reflux, depth of the GSV from skin (as noted on US), and presence of ulcer and multiple varicosities. A practical point to be remembered is that the introducer needle traverses at an angle from the skin entry site to reach the superficial vein.

The perforators may or may not be marked, depending on ultrasound operator's comfort level.

With the availability of sterile probe covers and ultrasound jellies, the lower extremities may be prepped and draped and, venous mapping using ultrasound performed subsequently.

Considering that the incompetent vein(s) were already identified on a diagnostic ultrasound, mapping includes localizing the highest and lowest point of reflux. The lowest point will guide in determining the site of skin entry. Identification of some key vein morphology is crucial to procedure. The tortuosity of vein needs to be recognized and it needs to be anticipated that how much of tortuosity would be appropriate for the guide wire to negotiate. There have been cases in our practice where extreme and humungous tortuosity of the main truncal vein has rendered the vein non-negotiable by guide-wire introduced via a single venous access. As a result, the sheath cannot be advanced to the targeted location. These cases have warranted a second access into the truncal vein, possibly above the site of tortuosity and then treat the vein in different segments. The intervening tortuosity can be managed with microphlebectomy or sclerotherapy.

The presence of aneurysmal segments in target vein needs to be recognized as well. For laser fibers to act effectively, the walls of these dilated venous segments need to be apposed i.e., closer to each other, or at least the laser fiber. During the procedure, these aneurysmal segments need special attention, as they segments may require additional laser energy for ablation.

The proximity of any nerves to the venous segment of the target vein to be treated is worth mentioning here. This particularly applies to segments of GSV and SSV, which are in proximity to saphenous and sural nerve, respectively.

The post thrombotic squeal in superficial vein can pose problems. One such condition is presence of post thrombotic webs within the venous lumen, which may offer obstruction to the passage of guide-wire.

Within the vein, laser energy has its effect on the structures located in vicinity of the laser fiber. The proponents of tumescent anesthesia have discussed this extensively. However, in situations when there is not much tissue adjoining the vein being treated, and the overlying skin is in close proximity to the vein, laser energy may damage the skin resulting in breakdown, thereby causing skin burn and ulceration. Tumescent bath is certainly of help in these conditions. Alternatively, if there is only one such segment of vein that is in skin's proximity, it may be left untreated with laser, but can be treated by instilling sclerosant. You can do that in the same sitting either by the same venous access (i.e., withdraw the laser fiber while keeping the sheath in place, with tip of the sheath located at inferior margin of vein segment you plan to leave untreated with laser, and then subsequently instill foamed sclerosant through the sheath into this segment. Having done that, you can introduce the laser fiber through the sheath and resume treating the veins segment that is at a suitable distance from the skin, with laser) or you can skip this segment which is closer to the skin, withdraw the fiber-sheath interlock and resume laser treatment in the vein segment which is suitable for treatment. You can access the intervening untreated segment separately and instill sclerosant in that.

Patient and table positioning

In our practice, we have performed procedures in supine positions, irrespective of type of anesthesia used. However, during some of the procedures we had to turn the patient partially to either side, either to gain access or trace a perforator and/or venous channel. For the most part supine has been the working position.

Sometimes reverse Trendelenburg position, wherein the feet level is 15-30 degrees below the head level, can be of help. This position encourages gravitational assisted pooling of venous blood in lower extremities, thereby making the leg veins prominent and easy for access. Additionally, the effectiveness of spinal or epidural anesthetic is increased, if that has been administered for the procedure. You may find this position particularly effective when performing procedure on an obese or morbidly obese individual.

In our set up, the laser-operating physician (Procedure physician or PP) preferred to be at the foot end of procedure table. The ultrasound-operating physician (UOP) in most cases, preferred to be on right side of the patient. The ultrasound machine usually stays on the side of ultrasound-operating physician due to ease of operability. Though, there have been instances wherein space constraints in the procedure room mandated placement of ultrasound machine across the procedure table, i.e., on the side opposite of ultrasound-operating physician. In such situations, UOP may require help from an individual, to operate the ultrasound machine keyboards. Depending on worldwide geographic location, the services of ultrasound technologist may be utilized instead of UOP.

The surgical table and laser machine position in the operating room is usually the laser-operating physician's preference. It should though be kept in mind that the laser fiber is sterile, whereas the laser machine base unit is not. During the procedure, when PP offers the laser fiber to an operating room staff, in order to attach fiber interlock to the laser base unit, the interlock system of fiber is no longer sterile. The overhanging portion of the fiber, extending from the interlock to the fiber tip, is sterile though, and hangs as a bridge from base unit table (on which laser base unit has been mounted) and the surgical table. Beyond this point in the procedure, any trespassing across the overhanging fiber within the operating room must be restricted. This is a key safety measure which needs to be observed, not only to maintain sterile state of laser fiber, but also preventing running into the thin, light colored laser fiber and inadvertently disrupting the fiber interlock with the base unit, and potentially hazardous and traumatic withdrawal of laser fiber from within the patient. **Note:** The laser fiber is not interlocked with the base at this initial time of procedure. We have mentioned about the fiber here at this stage of the chapter because it has an impact on positioning of the base unit table

The footplate of laser system which triggers laser firing is placed near either foot of the laser-performing physicians, whichever is preferred by this physician. Care should be maintained that this foot plate is not accessible to anybody else's foot, even inadvertently, else that could result in non-directed laser-fiber firing in undesired location, which could be within or outside the patient's body. Outside the patient's body the inadvertent laser firing is harmful to personnel present within the procedure at that time.

Prep & Drape

Prepping of lower extremity should include the infra-umbilical region of abdomen, respective groins, thighs, knee, legs, ankle and foot. It may be argued that the extent of prepping is excessive, considering the percutaneous approach, particularly when the venous access site is in the leg. But in our practice this has helped us in unexpected challenging situations. For example, situations when we could not advance laser fiber through the GSV in thigh region, additional venous access was necessitated in relatively central location in thigh.

While draping the lower extremity, it would be helpful to drape and cover the toes and leave the prepped ankle, forefoot and possibly mid foot open to access. Experiences and trained surgical assistants can be explained to prep as for cardiac bypass surgery (CABG), and that gives them a fair idea of what's required.

Care must be taken to drape the foot and leave the ankle as sterile open field in the event that GSV and/or perforators need be treated or accessed at that level.

Venous access

Following venous marking and sterile preparations, venous access at the chosen site is obtained. Of all the key steps involved in this procedure, we rate venous access as the strikingly important step, as the access to GSV serves the route for all the subsequent steps in this procedure.

A local anesthetic is administered in cutaneous and subcutaneous plane at the proposed skin entry site. It is essentially that all the air is removed from the needle and syringe used for local anesthetic administration, because presence of air within the subcutaneous tissue will obscure visualization of structures on ultrasound, and you invariably might have to choose another access site. Administering the local anesthetic under ultrasound guidance is a good idea, as you can see and estimate the require amount to be instilled. If you administer volume disproportionate to what the space can hold, chances are you will encounter an overlying skin bump, compression of underlying superficial vein which is your target, or may be both.

We have been using a 18-Gauge puncture needle in our practice, but basically whichever needle is used, make sure beforehand that the guide-wire goes through the access needle easily (the guide wire usually being 0.035 inches), since that would be the next logical step in this procedure.

Access into GSV is gained under US guidance. The choice of transducer placement along the transverse versus longitudinal axis of GSV is upon the UOP. Although, we have found both useful, we recommend getting comfortable with one or the other imaging plane first. The transverse plane, according to our experience is better since it provides information regarding side-to-side landing of introduced access needle, and at the same time allows localization and adjustment of needle entry into the anterior GSV wall in a craniocaudal plane.

The access needle should be advanced and localized onto the anterior GSV wall. Thereafter, under US guidance, the needle is introduced into the vein. The return of blood from the needle hub exteriorly is not the confirmation that needle tip is localized within the venous lumen. We have often found that advancing the needle a little beyond the posterior wall of GSV, and then pulling back the needle into the GSV lumen optimizes the path for subsequent guidewire advancement. For those who want to stick with anterior wall only, and still want to confirm their intraluminal location, can gently advance guidewire through the needle into the vein under US guidance, and see if it goes easily into the vein. If not, the guidewire should not be stirred or forced into the vein. It is advisable to withdraw the guidewire, lest the vein lands into spasm which makes further steps all the more difficult, and may also require abandoning this site for access.

Another point worth mentioning is the localization of access needle tip within the venous lumen. Logically it may seem that once you localize the tip within the anechoic lumen of the vein, the needle should be intraluminal. But that does not happen all the time, particularly if the vein is accessed using US probe in longitudinal dimension. Ultrasound beam, being in a real time plane may be traversing the nearby intimal

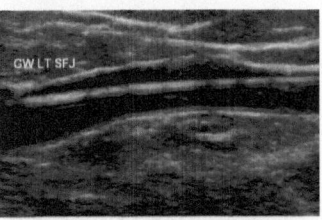

9.4 Image. Guidewire appearance on ultrasound

layer, middle lumen and distant intimal layer of the vein, all in one plane. Partial-volume effect could result in apparent localization of the needle tip within the lumen, when it actually may be in the nearby intima (or sub-intimal). There can be blood return from the needle hub even if the needle tip is sub-intimal plane. An experienced sonographer may be able to recognize the needle traversing the intima and entering lumen. The smooth passage of guidewire through the needle into the venous lumen is confirmatory though.

Endovenous procedure

Once the access into GSV has been obtained, a 0.035" guidewire is advanced through the introducer needle into the vein. The guidewire can be seen advancing into the vein under US, all the way tracing up to the SFJ. The guidewire appears as linear echogenic material within the vein, which has reverberation artifacts (see image 9.4).

Next, the introducing needle is withdrawn. A No.11 surgical blade is used to create a skin nick at the guidewire entrance site. This is made to minimize resistance provided by the skin to the passage of 5-Fr introducer sheath-dilator unit.

Next, the sheath-dilator system (typically 40 cm, but may be different with different systems) is advanced over the guidewire into the vein. The sheath can be seen advancing into the vein, over the guidewire under US, appearing as a double walled echo tubular structure (see images 9.5-9.10). Once the sheath-dilator system has been advanced all the way through its entire length, the

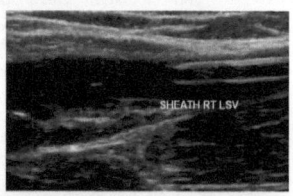

9.5 Image. Appropriate positioning of sheath in GSV

9.6 Image. Appearance of appropriate positioning of sheath

tip of sheath can be localized on US, which is usually in mid-thigh in an average height person, given that the venous access is in distal leg. Although the sheath-dilator system is advanced over the guide-wire, which was earlier introduced into the GSV, the intraluminal location of sheath-dilator system must not be assumed. The system may cause a kink in guide-wire, which can lead to curling a capacious vein. This then may also cause loss of already gained venous access in the proximal GSV and SFJ. Therefore, prior to removal of dilator from the sheath, intraluminal location of the sheath must be
confirmed. Following the intraluminal confirmation of sheath location, the dilator as well as the guide-wire can be withdrawn.

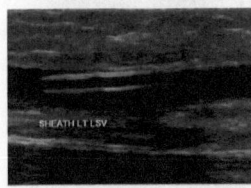

9.7 Image. Sheath positioning in a distended vein

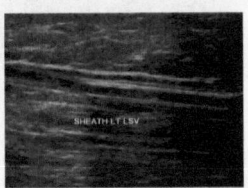

9.8 Image. Sheath appearance in a collapsed vein

We recommend that once location of sheath is confirmed, next step should be setting up the laser-fiber interlock with

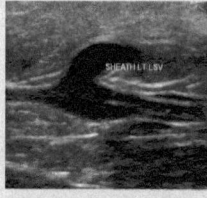
9.9 Image. Sheath position careful for fiber advancement

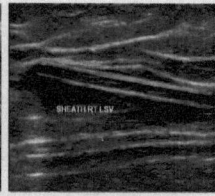
9.10 Image. Sheath position not appropriate

the laser base unit, and then withdraw dilator and guidewire. The reason being, setting up of fiber interlock may take couple of minutes, and in the meantime if the dilator and sheath have been withdrawn, the segment of vein beyond the sheath tip may collapse and/or thrombose, which can pose difficulty in advancing the fiber. In the event that happens, manipulating and advancing the laser-fiber in the vein may cause venous wall perforation, and the laser-fiber may land up in extra-luminal location. This is potentially possible when you expect the least resistance offered by surrounding perivenous fat in the groin or upper thigh region.

So, having confirmed the intraluminal location of sheath, establishing the laser-fiber interlock with base unit, and withdrawal of dilator and guide-wire, the firing tip end of fiber can then be through the sheath into the accessed vein. The advancing course of this fiber generally does not require US guidance up to known length of the sheath. For example, if the introduced sheath is 40 cm long, the fiber is expected to be within the sheath up to that length (40 cm in this case), prior to its exit through the sheath's distal tip. At that point it is wise to follow the course of fiber within the vein, under US guidance, as it is advanced towards the SFJ. The fiber appears as linear echogenic structure on US. The tip of fiber is advanced up to 2 – 2.5 cm peripheral to SFJ. In skinny patients, the localizer light of laser can be seen from outside, providing surface correlate of the intraluminal location.

It is very critical to that the fiber tip is outside the sheath margins before laser is fired, else the laser energy destroys the sheath and may leave fragments of it within the treated vein, which subsequently has potential for foreign body reaction and may also act as nidus for infection.

Locations of laser-fiber tip in relation to the SFJ

The initial practice was to position the fiber tip 1 cm peripheral to SFJ. Thereafter the trend has been to position the tip 2 cm peripheral to SFJ. Currently, a distance of 2.5 cm may be the preferred one. The increasing shift may be related to increasing awareness about Endothermal heat induced thrombosis (EHIT).

Thrombus formation in the superficial venous system is an expected outcome of endovenous laser or RF ablation. What really matters is the extent of this thrombus. EHIT has been described subsequently in post procedure outcomes chapter. Its relevance to SFJ-fiber tip distance is described here, as follows.

EHIT class I is described as thrombosis to the level of SFJ. EHIT class II refers to thrombus which extends from superficial system, crosses the SFJ and extends into the deep venous system, involving less than or equal to 50 % of the cross sectional area.

Increasing ablation distance peripheral to SFJ may result in diminished rate of EHIT, as reported by Sadek et al[1]. This article compared the incidence of EHIT following endovenous ablation procedures when the distance was increased from 2 cm to 2.5 cm and above. Reportedly, the incidence of EHIT in earlier studies was 16 % when distance was 1 cm, which then moved down to 4 % and then 2.3 % as the experienced hands increased along with the increase in distance from SFJ. Sadek et al reported the incidence of 1.3% when distance was kept at or above 2.5 cm.

Our experience with the distance has been no different. We have definitely stayed past 1 cm in our initial procedures. With increasing realization and understanding of EHIT, we preferred to stay in the range of 2 – 2.5 cm from SFJ. (see images 9.11-9.14).

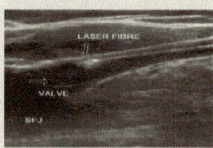
9.11 Image. Fiber positioning

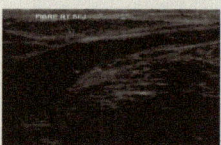
9.12 Image. Fiber position appropriate

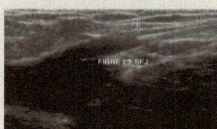
9.13 Image. Fiber position appropriate

9.14 Image. Laser fiber position not appropriate

The location of fiber tip within the GSV can be estimated by its laser glow that can be seen externally via translucent skin (see image 9.15). Ultrasound though is an accurate and handy tool we have to ascertain the exact location of fiber tip in relation with the SFJ.

Tumescent anesthesia

The meaning of "tumescent" is swollen. Tumescent anesthesia is the practice of injecting local anesthetic (combined with epinephrine and sodium bicarbonate) into the tissues that makes the tissue firm, tense and swollen[2,15]. Initially used in liposuction, this technique has potential uses in endovenous ablation. Extensive regional anesthesia of skin and subcutaneous tissue is achieved by subcutaneous infiltration of diluted lidocaine and epinephrine. Diluted epinephrine causes vasoconstriction, which diminishes the rate of systemic lidocaine absorption, permitting usage of large dose of lidocaine without systemic toxicity[3]. Epinephrine also reduces the incidence of hematoma and hyperpigmentation[19]. Bicarbonate diminishes the burning sensation from the injected local anesthesia, potentiates the anesthetic effect and reduces the amount required for desired effect[20].

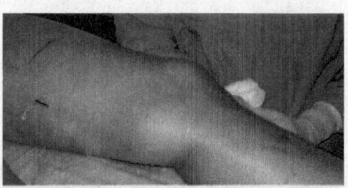

9.15 Image. Externally visible pilot light of laser fiber from within the vein

Solution contents: The solution was prepped during the procedure using approximately 500 ml of normal saline, 50 ml of 1 % lidocaine with epinephrine and 10 ml of 8.4 % sodium bicarbonate.

Mode of delivery: In our practice, we used hand injections of either 20 cc or 50 cc syringes and 21 G spinal needles. The anesthetic solution was delivered under US guidance around the GSV in which the sheath and laser fiber can be seen. The injecting needle is advanced in such a way so that the needle path is visualized by US beam. Needle is advanced to penetrate the saphenous fascia, and then the fluid is injected. (see image 9.16) The linear US transducers are usually 4-5 cm long, and therefore we injected sites along the marked GSV course every 5 cm.

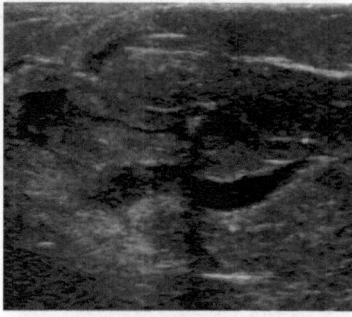

9.16 Image. Tumescent anesthesia in perivenous region surrounding laser fiber (in transverse section)

There however are various systems available which deliver this solution, one of it being the foot pump delivery system.

Role of tumescent anesthesia in endovenous ablation:

1. It creates a heat sink in perivenous space[16]. The peak temperature generated in the perivenous tissue during the endovenous laser is reduced with the use of perivenous tumescent fluid. The tumescent liquid also minimizes the number of venous wall perforations by the laser fiber, preventing perivenous tissue destruction[18].
2. Separates GSV from saphenous nerve, minimizing the risk for post-procedure paresthesia.
3. Compresses the underlying vein that is being treated, reducing its diameter and facilitating fiber-venous wall contact.

Problems associated with tumescent anesthesia:

In our practice, we found patients reporting disproportionate pain or discomfort at the puncture sites through which tumescent anesthesia was administered. To further evaluate this post-procedure concern, we administered unilateral tumescent anesthesia in selected patients undergoing bilateral procedure. Nearly all these patients complained of post-procedure disproportionate pain or discomfort at tumescent puncture sites, when compared to the non-injected site.

There have been reports of lidocaine use without epinephrine[4]. More recently procedures without the use of tumescent anesthesia have also been performed[17]. The elimination of tumescent infusion has reduced the procedure time, but not significantly changed primary closure rates, ecchymosis, and post-procedure GSV diameters[5-7].

Realign the procedure table

If a reverse trendelenburg position was applied to the procedure table, it can be reverted back to normal angulation, once the venous access has been gained. This allows partial exsanguination of vein, thereby less blood in the lumen that helps in efficient transmission of laser energy to the venous wall, as well as less volume of blood available for clotting. The thrombus burden is thus subsequently reduced in the treated vein.

Precautionary gear

Before starting the laser, it is recommended that everyone in the procedure room wear the protective eye gear.

Laser Watt setting

This is the most calculative part of the procedure, that although appears tricky in the beginning, can be standardized to suit comfort zone of the treating physicians

9.17 Image. Empty the dilated vein prior to laser activation

own, with experience. The concept one needs to understand is of linear endovenous energy density (LEED), the unit of which is Joules per cm (J/cm). This essentially means energy delivered per cm length of treated vein, and is interplay between the wattage used to deliver energy, the time duration over which laser energy was delivered, and the length of the vein that was treated. Two additional factors play an instrumental role, the laser beam wavelength (i.e., 810 nm, 940 nm, 980 nm, 1470 nm, etc.) and the mode of laser energy delivery (i.e., pulse versus continuous mode).

A study to evaluate factors influencing effectiveness of endovenous laser ablation was published, which concluded that LEED is the main determinant of successful GSV ablation, and neither of the patient factors (body mass index or GSV diameter) influence the outcome[8].

From practical standpoint, you would still need to know the appropriate wattage for an individual machine to produce the desired effect. The laser machine companies technical experts and application specialists would be able to guide you with that.

LASER ACTIVATION (see images 9.17- 9.21)

Once the laser-fiber has been adequately positioned, tumescent anesthesia applied and protective eyewear worn, the laser unit is ready to be activated. It would be wise step to check the fiber tip position in relation with SFJ once again, making sure it is 2 cm or more peripheral to the SFJ, and has not inadvertently entered the deep vein while tumescent anesthesia was being administered. Once in a while we have seen laser fiber entering the perivenous compartment in the interim period. Any excessive dilated target vein can be manually compressed to empty in order to have good apposition of venous wall to the fiber. (see image 9.17).

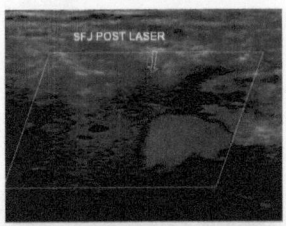
9.18 Image. Intra procedural SFJ post laser ablation

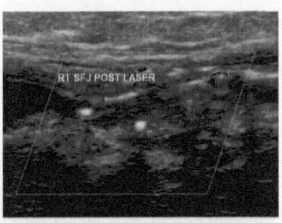
9.19 Image. Intra procedural SFJ post laser ablation

Having double-checked and verified the intraluminal location of fiber tip, laser can be activated using the foot pedal. Ultrasound performed simultaneously at the location overlying fiber tip demonstrates movement of blood and bubbles, emanating from the fiber tip. Echogenic areas can also be seen within the venous wall. The fiber is then withdrawn depending whether the pulse or continuous mode is used for laser energy delivery.

In a fairly straightforward incompetent GSV this may go smooth. With a thorough US assessment of vein prior to the procedure, one may not require ultrasound guidance for ablation and withdrawing component of the laser ablation. One may be able to localize the laser fiber tip by the pilot beam visible externally. However, it does not hurt to do this entire procedure under US guidance, and we personally have been doing that. US guidance becomes essential towards the terminal part of the ablation i.e. when the

9.20 Image. Intra procedural thigh GSV post laser ablation

laser fiber is nearing the skin entry site. You may not want to ablate the extra-venous tissue which is the soft tissue situated in between the venous entry site of the laser fiber and the skin entry site of fiber, since you may recall that the venous access was achieved at an angle, directed cranially.

For the duration when the laser fiber is firing (or activated as you may technically say), patients may feel discomfort, and describe a burning sensation at the site of treatment. This does not pose a problem when spinal anesthesia has been administered for the procedure purposes. But when performed under local anesthesia, it can be uncomfortable to patients, who then move their limbs during the procedure, which not only can interfere with sterility of the procedure field, but can also alter the fiber tip location within the vein. Personally, we have found pulse mode delivery better than continuous mode delivery of laser energy, for these patients. But one can always pause the ablation procedure for a few seconds or minutes, let the patient relax a bit, and then resume laser delivery.

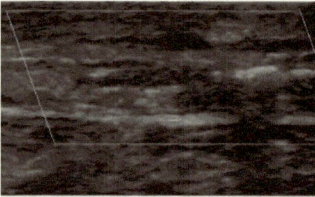

9.21 Image. Intra procedural leg GSV post laser ablation

Once the laser fiber is withdrawn completely out of the limb, a gentle compression using gauze over the skin entry site for a few seconds facilitates cessation of oozing.

Having ablated the truncal vein, one can direct attention towards treating other incompetent truncal vein by ablation, if that's the plan. The procedure basically remains the same, a repetition of the above mentioned procedure i.e., obtaining venous access, advancing guidewire and sheath successively, followed by introduction of laser fiber, which is then positioned at the highest point of reflux in the superficial vein (taking into the account the 2-2.5 cm distance to be kept from the superficial-deep vein junction to allow for junctional thrombus). Tumescent anesthesia is delivered along the course of this vein. The laser energy is adjusted according to vessel diameter, its proximity to the nerve, and distance from the skin. Laser is activated and fiber withdrawn, ablating the vein on its way.

At no point during the procedure should the fiber be landing into deep vein. Ultrasound can ascertain this anytime during the procedure. But, if the advancement of guidewire, sheath and laser fiber has been under US guidance, without entry into the deep vein, then the odds of laser tip landing in a deep vein while you are ablating the vein and withdrawing the fiber, are negligible (unless there has been unrecognized haywire positioning).

Endovenous Ablation of SSV
(see images 9.22 – 9.24)

If the SSV is known to be incompetent, and has been included in the ablation plan, it can be done at the same sitting as the other incompetent truncal vein being treated. In some patients, SSV could be the only incompetent vein that needs to ablation. In this latter scenario, patient positioning is different from what we have discussed above.

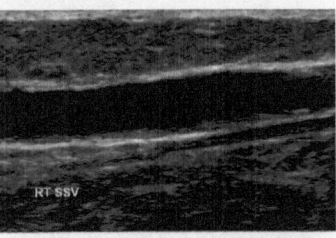

9.22 Image. Short saphenous vein pre-treatment

If SSV is the primary vein being treated, and there is no anteriorly located incompetent truncal vein to be ablated, then we have found prone patient position to be the best.

If SSV is one of the veins being treated, and there is other anteriorly located truncal vein to be treated, then beginning with routine supine position is recommended, albeit with a

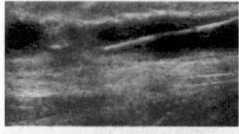
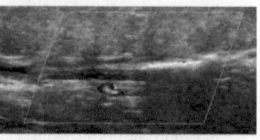

9.23 Image. Laser fiber in SSV at the time of ablation

9.24 Image. Intra procedural SSV post laser ablation

45-degree knee flexion of the extremity. This position helps in treating the GSV as well as the SSV. This has worked for us and one may try this. The other option is to change patient positioning once a vein has been ablated, but there are hurdles related to it, particularly the sterility of procedure field.

Besides positioning, the procedure otherwise is more or less the same. The venous access, and subsequent steps are the same. Due respect has to be given to the deep veins here as well, by staying away from them.

Endovenous ablation is effective in eliminating SSV reflux and providing symptomatic relief. Gibson et al reported that the incidence of nerve injury is low but the incidence of DVT was higher than the GSV ablation, and the anatomic features of SSV may predict the risk for developing DVT[9].

Varicosities and perforators

Once the main GSV and/or SSV and/or incompetent truncal tributaries have been ablated, there are different strategies to deal with varicosities and perforators.

Some believe in leaving them at the time of initial procedure, and evaluate them in follow up. If they persist, sclerotherapy may be performed to treat them. Others believe in performing laser ablation using laser fiber designed specifically for perforators. We have worked on concomitant use of endovenous laser for the main incompetent vein and sclerotherapy for tributaries and incompetent perforators. We presented our results at international platform and can be accessed in Journal of vascular and interventional radiology and Insights Imaging[10-14].

Features of this combined / concomitant therapy are:
- Safe
- Can be performed under local anesthesia as well
- Majority require no subsequent procedure
- If recurrence occurs, it's early in the post-treatment period.
- Markedly reduced symptoms
- Limits follow up clinic visits
- High acceptability of procedure amongst patients
- Avoids anxiety of undergoing procedures repeatedly.

The impact is social, economic and on time saved, as it limits the need of subsequent procedure.

Once the procedure is deemed complete, compression pads are applied over the venous access site(s). A grade II compression stocking is applied onto the treated limb.

Procedure-end imaging
The treatment end points on imaging include: venous wall damage evident by wall thickening, a reduction in vein diameter, and no flow on color and duplex exam

REFERENCES:

1. Sadek, Mikel et al. Increasing ablation distance peripheral to the saphenofemoral junction may result in a diminished rate of endothermal heat-induced

2. thrombosis. Journal of Vascular Surgery: Venous and Lymphatic Disorders, Volume 1 , Issue 3 , 257 - 262
2. 2. Patrick H. Conroy, James O'Rourke, Tumescent anaesthesia, The Surgeon, Volume 11, Issue 4, August 2013, Pages 210-221
3. 3. Klein JA. Tumescent technique for local anesthesia. Western Journal of Medicine. 1996;164(6):517.
4. 4. Hudson, A et al. Tumescent technique without epinephrine for endovenous laser therapy and serum lidocaine concentration. J Vasc Surg: Venous and Lym Dis 2015;3:48-53
5. 5. Korkmaz K, Yener AÜ, Selçuk Gedik H, et al. Tumescentless endovenous radiofrequency ablation with local hypothermia and compression technique. Cardiovascular Journal of Africa. 2013;24(8):313-317. doi:10.5830/CVJA-2013-053.
6. 6. Wright T F, Probst P J, Kennedy P (2012) Endovenous Laser Ablation without Tumescent Anesthesia. Cureus 4(11): e531.
7. 7. Osma, H. A comparative study of the efficacy of endovenous laser treatment of the incompetent great saphenous under general anesthesia with external air cooling with and without tumescent anesthesia. Dermatol Surg. 2013 Feb;39(2):255-62.
8. 8. N.S. Theivacumar, D. Dellagrammaticas, R.J. Beale, A.I.D. Mavor, M.J. Gough, Factors Influencing the Effectiveness of Endovenous Laser Ablation (EVLA) in the Treatment of Great Saphenous Vein Reflux, European Journal of Vascular and Endovascular Surgery, Volume 35, Issue 1, January 2008, Pages 119-123
9. 9. Gibson, Kathleen D. et al. Endovenous laser treatment of the short saphenous vein: Efficacy and complications. Journal of Vascular Surgery , 2007, 45 (4) : 795 - 803
10. 10. M.I. Bhalla, N. Bhalla. Treatment of lower limb varicosities with combined use of endovenous laser and sclerosant at the same instance - A unique study of 286 patients. Journal of Vascular and Interventional Radiology, Feb 2010; 21(2): S70

11. 11. M. Bhalla, N. Bhalla. Concomitant use of endovenous laser and foamed sclerosant for treatment of lower limb varicosities. Insights Imaging, 2011; 2(1): S275
12. 12. M.I. Bhalla, N. Bhalla. Concomitant use of endovenous laser and foamed sclerosant in the treatment of lower limb varicosities: 3 year follow-up results. Journal of Vascular and Interventional Radiology, 2011; 22(3): S18–S19
13. 13. M.I. Bhalla, N. Bhalla. Concomitant use of endovenous laser and foamed sclerosant in treatment of lower limb varicosities: 5 year follow-up results. Journal of Vascular and Interventional Radiology, March 2012; 23(3): S115
14. 14. M. Bhalla, N. Bhalla, H. Vasavada Concomitant use of endovenous laser and foamed sclerosant in treatment of lower limb varicosities: 3 year follow-up results. Insights Imaging, 2012; 3(1): S230
15. Memetoglu ME[1], Kurtcan S, Kalkan A, Özel D Combination technique of tumescent anesthesia during endovenous laser therapy of saphenous vein insufficiency. Interact Cardiovasc Thorac Surg. 2010 Dec;11(6):774-7
16. Zimmet SE[1], Min RJ. Temperature changes in perivenous tissue during endovenous laser treatment in a swine model. J Vasc Interv Radiol. 2003 Jul;14(7):911-5.
17. Hernández Osma E[1], Mordon SR, Marqa MF, Vokurka J, Trelles MA. A comparative study of the efficacy of endovenous laser treatment of the incompetent great saphenous under general anesthesia with external air cooling with and without tumescent anesthesia. Dermatol Surg. 2013 Feb;39(2):255-62
18. Vuylsteke, M.E. et al. Endovenous Laser Ablation: The Role of Intraluminal Blood. European Journal of Vascular and Endovascular Surgery , Volume 42 , Issue 1 , 120 – 126
19. Keel, D., Goldman, M.P. Tumescent anesthesia in ambulatory phlebectomy: addition of epinephrine. Dermatol Surg. 1999;25:371–372.

20. Klein, J.A. Anesthesia for liposuction in dermatologic surgery. J Dermatol Surg Oncol. 1988;14:1124–1132.

Chapter 10

SCLEROTHERAPY

Sclerosing means "abnormal hardening of body tissue". Sclerosant refers to injectable irritant material that causes venous intimal inflammation, subsequent fibrosis and lumen obliteration of vein. Sclerotherapy has been used for many years now, even in treatment of varicose veins. There are have been change in agents, mode of administration, and with development of endovenous ablation techniques, it has regained popularity as an adjunct method of treating varicose veins.

MECHANISM OF ACTION

Sclerosant, being osmotic agent and/or detergent causes endothelial damage. While the osmotic agents dehydrate endothelial cells through osmosis, the detergents interfere with cell membrane lipids thereby damaging the endothelium[10]. The procoagulant and anticoagulant activities of detergents have been shown in vitro[11].

INDICATIONS

1. Incompetent perforators.
2. Incompetent superficial truncal veins (including GSV and SSV).
3. Reticular veins.
4. Telangiectasia.
5. Recurrent venous bleeding.

Sclerosant can theoretically be injected in any incompetent superficial vein or perforator, but an understanding of the concept and the results this technique yields, is much more important to customize approach in individual patients.

Patients with venous ulceration are associated with more calf perforators compared to uncomplicated varicose veins. They may additionally be associated with deep venous reflux, which for obvious reasons is not our target for laser or sclerotherapy. However, treatment of incompetent perforators is necessary to minimize recurrence of this condition, and to have better clinical outcomes. While perforator surgery has been practiced for long, there are less invasive options available currently. Dedicated endovenous laser fibers for perforators are available which have been exclusively designed to ablate the incompetent perforators.

In patients having concomitant superficial and perforator incompetence, treating only the superficial system may not be correct the perforator incompetence. Intuitive as it may sound, the removal of abnormal superficial truncal vein may not do anything to stop the outflow of high-pressure venous blood through the perforator towards the skin vasculature. Direct surgical management of perforator by SEPS is definitive, but only for that particular perforator. Multiple such incompetent perforators need to be dealt with individually.

Sclerosant has an advantage over surgery. When injected through one venous access site, it can flow in the superficial veins and multiple adjoining perforators, thereby sclerosing the venous channels and causing occlusion of most of them. By the same logic, one needs to keep in mind, that the injected sclerosant makes its way into the deep veins of the lower extremity and thereby into the systemic circulation, both the locations where you would not want to have its potential effect.

While a bleeding varicosity requires acute management, the recurring condition can be managed with sclerotherapy.[2,3]

CONTRAINDICATIONS
Absolute contraindication: Acute thrombophlebitis.

Relative contraindication:
1. Pregnant patients.
2. History of migraine.
3. Patent foramen ovale – there is risk for microembolism[4-9]. Transient neurologic complications (visual disturbances and confusion) have been reported.
4. Ankle brachial index < 0.9 (peripheral vascular disease; DM) – there are risks for wound complications.

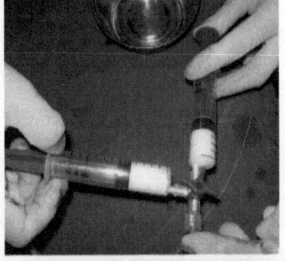
10.1 Image. Tessari technique for foam preparation

Concerning events with sclerotherapy:

A very few percentage of patients are reported to have adverse events. For example, in an article reported by Gillet et al, out of 1025 patients who underwent sclerotherapy, 8 (0.78%) had migraine, 7 (0.68%) had visual disturbances, 7 (0.68%) had chest pressure, and 1 (0.1%) had transient ischemic event[5].

AVAILABLE SCLEROSANTS

- Sodium tetradecyl suflate
- Polidocanol
- Glycerine
- Hypertonic saline

Different institutions have different preferences for sclerosant, and all of them are comparable[12,13]. In our practice, we have used sodium tetradecyl sulfate and polidocanol. Both of these are available in different concentrations, and need to be diluted prior to injecting.

PREPARATIONS: LIQUID VERSUS FOAM

Diluted liquid sclerosant is used as such in diluted format. The volume however depends upon the caliber and length of vein being treated.

Foam has the advantage of its geometric spherical shape. A sphere has a larger surface area, and therefore a foamed sclerosant has a larger potential area of contact with the vein wall. This has two key advantages: the amount of sclerosant used to achieve a desired effect, is less compared to the amount used in liquid form, and its more effective on larger caliber veins. The liquid sclerosant wash out is relatively quick, inducing relatively less vasospasm and sclerosing effect compared to foam[31].

FOAM PREPARAING TECHNIQUE (see image 10.1)

Tessari's technique is a simple method of preparing foam, using air and diluted sclerosant mixture, by two syringes and a three way stop cock. Additionally, there has been several other foam preparing techniques described in literature[14-18]. Alternatively, there are dispensers available which mix the gas and sclerosant to provide foamed mixture. In our practice, we have exclusively used the hand technique described by Tessari.

Two syringes (5 mL and/or 10 mL), one filled with air, and the other filled with a diluted sclerosant, are connected using a three-way. Practitioners of sclerotherapy have described using several different dilutions of sclerosant. In our practice, we used 1:2 to 1:4 dilution (i.e., 1mL of sclerosant and 2mL to 4mL of sterile normal saline). It is preferable to obtain the resultant foam in a 5 mL syringe since those are physically easier to inject through the needle into the vein. The aperture of 3-way is kept partially open, and the mixture then oscillated between the syringes to produce smooth foam.

Shelf life of foam: The foam should be prepared immediately prior to use, preferably within a minute. The half-life of foam prepared by Tessari technique is 90 seconds.

ULTRASOUND GUIDED FOAM SCLEROTHERAPY (UGFS) TECHNIQUE

Ultrasound

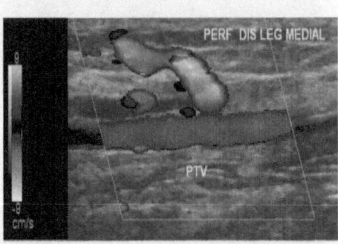

10.2 Image. Ultrasound demonstration of competent perforator draining into deep vein of leg. Note the color invert settings

Ultrasound guidance is the key component of this procedure as well. It is required for localizing the venous channels to be treated, guidance for gaining venous access, to monitor passage of sclerosant within the veins, and to ensure the resulting effects on vein. Typically, a linear array, high frequency transducer is required (we used 10-12 MHz linear transducer). However, in patients with grossly edematous and swollen legs, we had to switch to a 5-7 Mhz probe, to gain depth resolution. Ultrasound settings need to be optimum prior to procedure (see image 10.2). A pre-treatment planning measurement is performed for assessing the depth of perforators fascial penetration, and its distance from the skin. (see images 10.3-10.5)

Procedural preparations.

Since the half of foamed sclerosant is too short, it's practically very beneficial to set up everything you would require, on the tray beforehand. In a typical procedure you would have prepped the treating part in a sterile fashion (in sclerotherapy performed concomitant to the laser therapy, you might have done that already). The ultrasound probe has to be prepped in a sterile fashion. On the procedure tray,

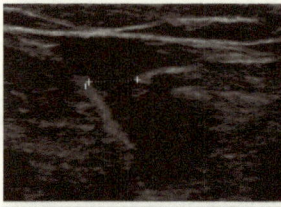

10.4 Image. Pre sclerotherapy perforator

10.3 Image. Pre-treatment planning for perforator

the required items include 5 and 10 mL syringes (at least 2-3), 24 Gauge needle (for sclerosant injection), 21 Gauge needle (if you want to aspirate sclerosant from the vial; we just had the vial contents dropped into the sterile bowl on the tray), a three way, normal saline, and some gauze pieces.

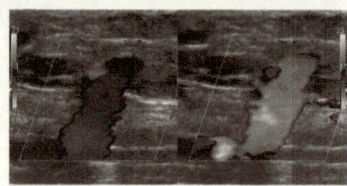

10.5 Image. Incompetent perforator pre-treatment

Administering sclerosant

Presuming that the incompetent veins have been mapped out earlier, they are localized under ultrasound. We preferred the initial injection in most caudal incompetent perforator or superficial venous channel, as the sclerosant would have a chance to proceed with antegrade venous flow and enter various channels and perforators on its way. This could potentially save multiple injections, reduce the total amount of sclerosant required for treatment, and reduce patient discomfort.

A 24 G needle is then advanced under US guidance until its deep is seen within the target vein. The targeted location within a superficial vein is most caudal segment, and in a perforator is the superficial component of the perforator (the segment that is situated superficial to the muscular fascia, or even a superficial channel that leads to this perforator). Once the blood return at the needle hub is verified, the syringe containing foamed sclerosant is attached to this 24 G needle. This can be a tricky step in this procedure, since you may not want the needle tip dislodging from the targeted location towards either side, i.e., either outside of the vein or into deeper component of the perforator. An alternative to this is connecting the syringe to needle prior to introducing across skin. If you apply this technique, the blood return from the vein can be verified by aspirating through the syringe before the sclerosant is injected.

In any approach you take, the aim is to deliver the foamed sclerosant into the target vein, which can be seen on ultrasound as dirty echogenic mobile echoes which results from tiny air bubbles within the foam (see images 10.6 and 10.7). The echogenic material can be seen advancing into the superficial vein and perforators. Some physicians believe in raising the leg to get anti-gravity support and empty the veins, but that is debatable and not practiced by all. The sclerosant invariably reaches the deep veins in few seconds. At this point, patient can be asked to perform few ankle dorsiflexion maneuver's that can help clear the sclerosant from deep vein.

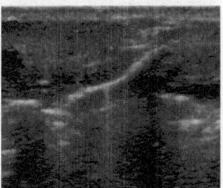

10.6 Image. Linear echogenic appearance with dirty shadowing in the region of previously identified incompetent perforator. Typical appearance of sclerosant on ultrasound.

Although theoretically this sclerosant can induce DVT, the incidence is not seen practically, not in our practice, and also worldwide. It may be because the compression stockings that are applied following sclerotherapy appose the superficial vein walls when the sclerosant has already had a chance to act on them, but the deep veins are not affected by that compression.

Careful: Stop injecting if at any point the foam is seen in extra-venous space. One, it will obscure evaluation of the target vein, possibly inducing spasm, thereby rendering it a less discernable target. Two, it will cause inflammation in perivenous space, which has the potential of fibrosis and scarring that can induce pain and discomfort, and can also cause discoloration of soft tissue.

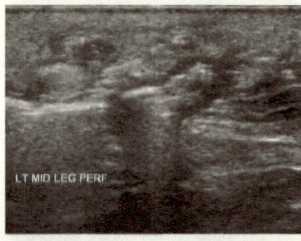

10.7 Image. Intraprocedural sclerosant in perforator and adjoining superficial varicosities

Amount of sclerosant: There have been differing numbers published on the total amount of sclerosant that can be injected safely, and individual amount that can be injected in each superficial vein[19]. Fortunately, with foam, not much is required. However, it is not advisable to inject > 10mL[30,34]. In our practice the maximum we required to inject was 6mL. If this procedure is being performed for incompetent perforators, in the same sitting as endovenous laser for truncal vein, then the amount is understandably even lower.

The procedure may be repeated for different (incompetent) perforators and superficial veins under ultrasound guidance, as the foam from initial injection may not have reached some channels in sufficient amount. While the leg perforators, superficial veins and even SSV can be treated in similar fashion, the thigh perforators and additional incompetent venous channels may require a longer and wider access needle, and relatively slight more amount of foam.

POST SCLEROTHERAPY COMPRESSION

Once the sclerotherapy is complete, bandage rolls are applied over the treated leg. Applying crepe bandage or straight away grade 2 compression stockings, over the bandage rolls can provide compression. In our practice, we ultimately had the patient wear grade 2 stockings, say for example, within 2-3 days of the procedure. Immediately after the procedure, we preferred applying crepe bandage. The intention behind having bandage rolls applied to the treated site is to reduce the friction between crepe bandage and treated site, and possibly reduced the skin discoloration and thrombophlebitis. Crepe bandages applied earlier on following the procedure are kept in place for 2 days, following which patient can remove and check for any skin changes. Thereafter, patient can switch to using grade 2 compression stockings. By no means should the crepe bandage be used beyond 2-3 days as their effect weans off over time, thereby voiding the desired compression effect. Exceptions are the conditions, which preclude wearing compression stockings in a recommended manner, for example leg ulcer. In such cases, patient can use crepe bandage as a means for compression, but needs to change to a new set every few days.

In treatment of telangiectasia's, 3 weeks of compression has shown improved cosmetic outcomes compared to those who had no or < 3 weeks post sclerotherapy compression, with correlation noted between the duration of compression and the degree of improvement[27-29].

EFFECTIVENESS OF FOAM SCLEROTHERAPY

There are numerous ways that sclerotherapy can be performed, either as an individual procedure, or in combination with other treatment modalities. Not surprisingly, there are varying results worldwide. We would like to summarize our experience.

1. Foam sclerotherapy is an excellent approach for incompetent perforators, particularly in patients with venous ulcers. If these patients have GSV and/or SSV incompetence, we treated these truncal veins with endovenous laser, and concomitantly treated the perforators with sclerotherapy (i.e. in the same treatment session). Ulcer healing with UGFS is comparable to surgery, with healing rate of 79% and 96% at one and three months, respectively[24-26]. (see images 10.8 and 10.9).

2. If the perforator incompetence is isolated I.e., without truncal incompetence, then we have exclusively used sclerotherapy. UDFS is very effective approach in treating perforator reflux, with a reported closure rate of 98% initially, and 75% at 5 years[23].

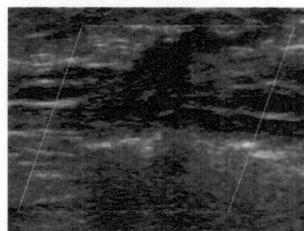

10.8 Image. Post sclerotherapy perforator

3. Foam sclerotherapy is very efficient procedure in cases of recurrence when incompetence is detected only in perforators.

4. We have tried sclerotherapy, as an individual procedure for GSV and SSV, in patients who due to varied reasons preferred this procedure to endovenous laser. The short-term results (6 months to 1 year) could be comparable to laser but the long-term results are clearly poor[20-22]. Given the choice, we would not prefer this for treatment of GSV, except procrastinating laser treatment is the goal. Sclerotherapy for isolated SSV incompetence may be performed, and we have had intermediate results with that, however, repeated sclerotherapy sessions yield better results. As a representative example,

GSV closure rate with endovenous laser was 93% compared to 77% with foam sclerotherapy[20].

POST SCLEROTHERAPY EXPECTED EVENTS AND POSSIBLE COMPLICATIONS

Some of the expected outcomes following sclerotherapy are: phlebitis related pain, localized swelling and discoloration. Phlebitis is the most common complain, which can be managed with analgesics and compression bandage/ stocking. The incidence can vary with the concentration of used sclerosant[32]. Intense superficial thrombophlebitis could be bothersome to the patient, and may need aspiration of thrombus under ultrasound guidance.

Discoloration or hyperpigmentation can develop within few days of the procedure, that spontaneously resolves in most of the patients, over a period that may extend to 2 years[33].

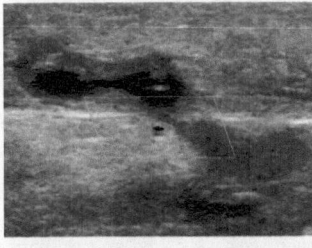

10.9 Image. Post sclerotherapy perforator

Localized swelling can be inflammatory response, which reduces with compression stockings and anti-inflammatory medications. Depending upon the pre-treatment caliber and proximity to the skin, the sclerosed and thrombosed treated superficial vein may have a feeling of lump, which may take few months to regress. Compression stocking is helpful in these conditions as well, however treating physicians have tried microphlebectomy of these veins, which itself is associated with scarring and discomfort.

Possible complications include deep venous thrombosis, and the events described under relative contraindication section above. With careful hands and ultrasound guidance, the incidence of DVT is very low, down to 1.7 % as reported in a large series of patients[34].

Endovenous foam-induced thrombus (EFIT) is equivalent of EHIT seen post-endothermal ablation, described later in chapter 12, and is managed in same manner, as EHIT.

REFERENCES:

1. Stuart WP, Adam DJ, Allan PL, Ruckley CV, Bradbury AW. Saphenous surgery does not correct perforator incompetence in the presence of deep venous reflux. J Vasc Surg 1998;28:834-8.
2. Labas P, Cambal M. Profuse bleeding in patients with chronic venous insufficiency. Int Angiol 2007; 26:64.
3. Hamahata A, Yamaki T, Osada A, et al. Foam sclerotherapy for spouting haemorrhage in patients with varicose veins. Eur J Vasc Endovasc Surg 2011; 41:856.
4. Forlee MV, Grouden M, Moore DJ, Shanik G. Stroke after varicose vein foam injection sclerotherapy. J Vasc Surg 2006; 43:162.
5. Gillet JL, Guedes JM, Guex JJ, et al. Side-effects and complications of foam sclerotherapy of the great and small saphenous veins: a controlled multicentre prospective study including 1,025 patients. Phlebology 2009; 24:131.
6. Hartmann, K. Reversible neurologic deficit after foam sclerotherapy. Eur J Vasc Endovasc Surg 2009; Epub ahead of print.
7. Raymond-Martimbeau P. Transient adverse events positively associated with patent foramen ovale after ultrasound-guided foam sclerotherapy. Phlebology 2009; 24:114.

8. Ceulen RP, Sommer A, Vernooy K. Microembolism during foam sclerotherapy of varicose veins. N Engl J Med 2008; 358:1525.
9. Hanisch F, Müller T, Krivokuca M, Winterholler M. Stroke following variceal sclerotherapy. Eur J Med Res 2004; 9:282.
10. Goldman MP. Treatment of varicose and telangiectatic leg veins: double-blind prospective comparative trial between aethoxyskerol and sotradecol. Dermatol Surg 2002; 28:52.
11. Parsi K, Exner T, Connor DE, et al. In vitro effects of detergent sclerosants on coagulation, platelets and microparticles. Eur J Vasc Endovasc Surg 2007; 34:731.
12. Tisi PV, Beverley C, Rees A. Injection sclerotherapy for varicose veins. Cochrane Database Syst Rev 2006; :CD001732.
13. Schwartz L, Maxwell H. Sclerotherapy for lower limb telangiectasias. Cochrane Database Syst Rev 2011; :CD008826.
14. Monfreux A. Traitement scle´rosant des troncs saphe`nies et leurs collate´rales de gros calibre par le me´thode mus. Phle´bologie 1997;50:351–3
15. 14 Sadoun S, Benigni JP. The treatment of varicosities and tel- angiectases with TDS and Lauromacrogol foam. XIII World Congress of Phlebology, 1998. Conrad P, Myers K, eds. Abstract book. International Union of Phlebology, Sydney, 1998
16. 15 Tessari L. Nouvelle technique d'obtention de la scle´ro- mousse. Phle´bologie 2000;53:129
17. 16 Frullini A. New technique in producing sclerosing foam in a disposable syringe. Derm Surg 2000;26:705–6
18. 17 Flu¨ckinger P. Nicht-operative retrograde Varizenvero¨ - dung mit Varsylschaum. Schweizer Med Wochenschrift 1956;86:1368 – 70
19. P Coleridge Smith. Foam and liquid sclerotherapy for varicose veins. Phlebology,2009; 24(1): 62-72.
20. Gonzalez-Zeh R, Armisen R, Barahona S. Endovenous laser and echo-guided foam ablation in

great saphenous vein reflux: one-year follow-up results. J Vasc Surg 2008; 48:940.
21. Weiss RA, Munavalli G. Endovenous ablation of truncal veins. Semin Cutan Med Surg 2005; 24:193.
22. Goldman MP. Intravascular lasers in the treatment of varicose veins. J Cosmet Dermatol 2004; 3:162.
23. Masuda EM, Kessler DM, Lurie F, et al. The effect of ultrasound-guided sclerotherapy of incompetent perforator veins on venous clinical severity and disability scores. J Vasc Surg 2006; 43:551.
24. Nael R, Rathbun S. Effectiveness of foam sclerotherapy for the treatment of varicose veins. Vasc Med 2010; 15:27.
25. Pang KH, Bate GR, Darvall KA, et al. Healing and recurrence rates following ultrasound-guided foam sclerotherapy of superficial venous reflux in patients with chronic venous ulceration. Eur J Vasc Endovasc Surg 2010; 40:790.
26. Darvall KA, Bate GR, Adam DJ, et al. Ultrasound-guided foam sclerotherapy for the treatment of chronic venous ulceration: a preliminary study. Eur J Vasc Endovasc Surg 2009; 38:764.
27. Kern P, Ramelet AA, Wütschert R, Hayoz D. Compression after sclerotherapy for telangiectasias and reticular leg veins: a randomized controlled study. J Vasc Surg 2007; 45:1212.
28. Weiss RA, Sadick NS, Goldman MP, Weiss MA. Post-sclerotherapy compression: controlled comparative study of duration of compression and its effects on clinical outcome. Dermatol Surg 1999; 25:105.
29. Nootheti PK, Cadag KM, Magpantay A, Goldman MP. Efficacy of graduated compression stockings for an additional 3 weeks after sclerotherapy treatment of reticular and telangiectatic leg veins. Dermatol Surg 2009; 35:53.
30. Breu FX, Guggenbichler S, Wollmann JC. 2nd European Consensus Meeting on Foam Sclerotherapy 2006, Tegernsee, Germany. *Vasa* 2008; 37(Suppl 71): 1–29.

31. Hamel-Desnos C, Desnos P, Wollmann JC, Ouvry P, Mako S, Allaert FA. Evaluation of the efficacy of polidocanol in the form of foam compared with liquid form in sclerotherapy of the greater saphenous vein: initial results. Dermatol Surg 2003;29:1170-5
32. Blaise S, Bosson JL, Diamand JM. Ultrasound-guided sclerotherapy of the great saphenous vein with 1% *versus* 3% polidocanol foam: a multicentre double-blind randomized trial with 3-year follow-up. *Eur J Vasc Endovasc Surg* 2010;39: 779–786.
33. Goldman MP, Kaplan RP, Duffy DM. Postsclerotherapy hyperpigmentation: a histologic evaluation. J Dermatol Surg Oncol 1987; 13:547.
34. Kulkarni et al. The incidence and characterization of deep vein thrombosis following ultrasound-guided foam sclerotherapy in 1000 legs with superficial venous reflux. J Vasc Surg: Venous and Lym Dis 2013;1:231-8.

Chapter 11

POST PROCEDURE MANAGEMENT AND FOLLOW UP

PROCEDURE END

<u>Clean and compress</u>

Adequate and proper compression is vital following any procedure performed for venous insufficiency. Compression is highly effective in reducing postoperative bruising and tenderness, and can theoretically reduce the risk venous thromboembolism.

Once the ablation component of the procedure is completed, the treated limb is cleaned and dried. Small gauze is placed at the skin entry site of laser fiber. If endovenous laser is the only procedure that was performed, a class II compression stocking is applied to the treated limb right away. Now, if there is an ulcer and/or sclerotherapy performed in that limb, the application needs to be modified, depending upon the extent of ulceration. If the ulcer involves a dominant portion of leg, we apply crepe bandage to non-ulcerated portion of the limb, and sterile dressing over the ulcer. As mentioned in the previous chapter on sclerotherapy, elastic crape bandages are not an effective means of compression, but can be used up to 2-3 days following the procedure, under certain circumstances. Compression stockings are then recommended for at least 3 weeks.

A class II compression stocking provides a compression pressure of 30 mm Hg, and also needs to compress the treated thigh portion.

Treatment record

During the follow up visits, recall of a case specifics are much easier if the records of procedure are available, preferable in a visual format (like a diagram and/or chart). The details you may find useful are:
- Initial US findings and map of incompetent veins.
- Site of venous access for endovenous laser ablation of GSV and /or SSV.
- Length of treated GSV and/or SSV.
- Laser treatment: Watts used, total energy applied in Joules, total lasing time, pulse or continuous mode of laser delivery.
- Sclerotherapy: The agent used, its concentration, dilution and air mixture, and perforators treated.

IMMEDIATE POST PROCEDURE

1. Ambulate: Patients who had the procedure under local anesthesia are encouraged to ambulate immediately following the procedure. Each patient may vary individually depending upon the comfort level, but the idea is to get the blood moving in competent lower extremity veins. Those who have procedure under spinal anesthesia, are initially transported to recovery area, but are encouraged to ambulate when they are out of anesthetic effect, and when its deemed appropriate to walk. In our practice,

the norm was to oversee patient walk in the hospital corridor and then walk out of the hospital door at discharge. This instills confidence in patients, relatives and treating team.
2. Prescribe analgesics and/or anti-inflammatory for approximately 1 week.
3. Set follow-up clinic visits.

Role of LMW heparin:
Counterintuitive as it may seem, some treating physicians routinely recommend LMW heparin following the ablation procedure[1]. In our practice, we did not prescribe post-procedure heparin routinely, and so do not many physicians worldwide.

INSTRUCTIONS ON DISCHARGE
1. Wear stockings during the daytime.
2. Elevate legs (possibly by placing pillows underneath foot) while in bed.
3. Return to routine activities and work.
4. Avoid non-habitual strenuous activities for 1 week.
5. Keep the legs clean and dry.
6. Regular sterile dressing of ulcers.
7. Appropriate management of associated health conditions.
8. Start calf exercise regime.
9. Call back if warning signs or unexpected outcomes are noted.
10. Comply with follow-up clinic visits.

INTERMEDIATE AND LONG TERM GOAL

Beyond the time frame of few weeks from the ablation and/or sclerotherapy procedure, the goal is to capitalize on the benefits of treatment, and prevent its recurrence. Patients need to understand the underlying pathophysiology of venous insufficiency, and take appropriate measures for

long-term effectiveness of these procedures. Some of these are outlined below.
1. Improving overall health and well being of an individual.
2. Body weight and body mass index (BMI) to be within limits appropriate for age.
3. Strengthen muscle pump by calf exercises.

FOLLOW UP CLINIC VISITS

Schedule

The idea is to set up regular follow up and identify signs of recurrence early on. This may vary for every individual based on several factors, for example, the distance a patient travels to visit clinic, individual's profession, baseline extent of disease prior to treatment, etc. Yet, having a timeline listed on paper promotes compliance.

On an average, follow up at 2 weeks, 6 weeks, 3 months, 6 months and 12 months following the procedure, may work fine. But this needs to flexible enough, since there may be recurrence or repeats sessions of treatment required in between, or may be no intervening measures required at all.

Tasks for follow up visits
1. Clinical assessment, including symptomatology, following treatment. There may have been improvement, resolution, or transient worsening of symptoms. Ask for any new symptoms.
2. Ask for compliance with compression stockings and calf exercises.
3. Assess healing of ulcer and /or thrombophlebitis, and if appropriate sterile regular dressing of ulcer is being managed.
4. Ultrasound exam: This will assess for deep vein patency and reflux, ablation of superficial veins, sclerosed superficial channels and perforators, and new incompetent veins.
5. Repeat sclerotherapy of there is persistent reflux or new few incompetent perforators.

6. Photograph of treated limb.

What to look for
- Varicosities, skin changes, and ulceration
- Nerve injuries
- Level of extremity discomfort compared to pre-procedure

ULTRASOUND APPEARANCE OF TREATED VEIN

Laser ablation: Early on the venous wall appears thickened, intermittently echogenic and irregular. Intermediate echoes are seen within the lumen suggesting thrombosis. The caliber is reduced compared to pre-procedure imaging, and the vein is non-compressible. No color flow is identified within the lumen.

Further away from the procedure date, the vein appears fibrosed and may appear and thin echogenic strand or cord. Don't be surprised if you do not see any of the treated vein on long term follow up, as we have encountered such cases.

Sclerotherapy: The treated superficial channels and perforators show intermediate level echoes within it, suggesting thrombus. No color flow is seen. The superficial channels are non-compressible.

What to look for
- DVT
- Treated vein
- Any new incompetent vein / perforator
- EHIT

Defining occlusive thrombus: When the vein is completely filled by an incompressible, hypoechoic mass with no fluxes within the vessel lumen.

EHIT: Distance of central end of thrombus is measured from the SFJ. If the thrombus extends into deep vein, then the cross-sectional area of venous lumen affected by the lumen is assessed.

NOTE: Partial recanalization of vein can be seen, but the clinical significance is uncertain especially if the symptoms do not recur[3].

DEFINING OUTCOME MEASURES

Primary successful outcome measures
1. Anatomic success: occlusion of the treated vein.
2. Clinical success: improvement in VCSS.
3. Technical success: No technical problem in the planned procedure.

Secondary successful outcome measures
1. Post-procedural symptomatology, particularly pain.
2. Post-procedural complications, related to endovenous ablation or sclerotherapy.
3. Return to work and routine activities.
4. Overall improvement in quality of life.

Primary treatment failure
➢ Absence of wall changes or presence of reflux in treated vein.

Secondary treatment failure
➢ 10 cm recanalized treated vein segment (GSV)

POST-OPERATIVE HEMODYNAMIC CHANGES FOLLOWING ENDOVENOUS LASER ABLATION

Park et al reported the hemodynamic changes following endovenous laser ablation. The hemodynamic variables they evaluated were venous volume (VV), venous filling index (VFI), residual volume fraction (RVF), and ejection fraction (EF). These variables were evaluated pre-procedure and at 1 and 6 months post procedure[2].

All the hemodynamic variables improved following endovenous laser ablation. The VV, VFI and RVF decreased and EF increased. The only statistically significant improvement at 6 month compared to 1-month follow up was the EF, which increased further at 6 months, which expectedly might be due to improvement in calf function over time. Understandably, the VV which is related to the volume of GSV, and VFI and RVF which are related to the refluxing GSV, these parameters improved immediately with ablation of the GSV.

REFERENCES:

1. Proebstle, T.M. et al. Endovenous treatment of the greater saphenous vein with a 940-nm diode laser: Thrombotic occlusion after endoluminal thermal damage by laser-generated steam bubbles. Journal of Vascular Surgery 2002, 35 (4): 729 - 736
2. Park Y, Young-Wook Kim,Yang-Jin Park, et al.Postoperative hemodynamic changes after endovenous laser ablation and phlebectomy in varicose vein surgery.(J Vasc Surg: Venous and Lym Dis 2015;3:54-7.)
3. Gibson KD, Ferris BL, Polissar N,Neradilek B, Pepper D. Endovenous laser treatment of the short saphenous vein: efficacy and complications. J Vasc Surg 2007; 45:795– 801.

Chapter 12

EXPECTED OUTCOMES, RESULTS AND POSSIBLE COMPLICATIONS

The most frequent complain after the procedure, which in fact is an expected outcome, is the pain and/or soreness along the length of treated vein. This weans off over time, and may require anti-inflammatory or analgesics medications. Patient needs to be reassured that this is an expected symptom. Ultrasound appearance of ablated vein is reassuring as is the improvement in ulcer. (see images 12.1-12.6).

Mild increase edema is expected, particularly when a perivenous bath was created. An extremely edematous and painful extremity, however, should raise the concern for DVT. Comparing the limb diameter with a baseline measurement can be useful in such situations.

Ecchymosis can be caused by laser induced venous wall perforation. It is typically seen along the inner thigh and knee region, usually the day following the procedure, but can be noted even 2 weeks later. The findings are not as pronounced as could be seen with surgery.

In 2-3 weeks following laser ablation, patient may describe feeling of tightness and palpable induration along the length of treated vein, which can cause moderate pain when the limb is extended.

Hematoma can occasionally occur at any site along the vein, due to various reasons. Nothing in particular requires to be done for this. Analgesics/ anti-inflammatory medications, cold/warm compresses and compression stocking are helpful. This was a rare finding in our practice.

Superficial thrombophlebitis can develop anywhere along the treated length of the vein, particularly when sclerosant has been used. Puggioni et al reported an increased rate of painful thrombophlebitis and cellulitis with the endovenous laser ablation compared to the radiofrequency ablation[20]. The authors attributed this fact to an incomplete vein emptying, with intraluminal thrombus and surrounding inflammation.

Hyperpigmentation can occur along the overlying ablated GSV, but is relatively more common with sclerotherapy.

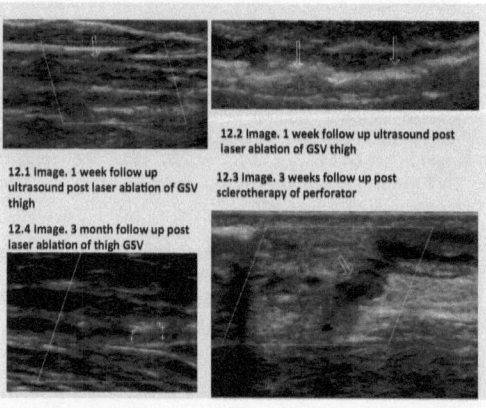

12.1 Image. 1 week follow up ultrasound post laser ablation of GSV thigh

12.2 Image. 1 week follow up ultrasound post laser ablation of GSV thigh

12.3 Image. 3 weeks follow up post sclerotherapy of perforator

12.4 Image. 3 month follow up post laser ablation of thigh GSV

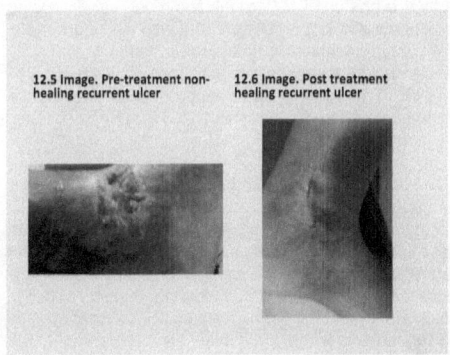

12.5 Image. Pre-treatment non-healing recurrent ulcer

12.6 Image. Post treatment healing recurrent ulcer

NOTE:
1. Patient needs to be instructed that any of the expected outcomes should not limit the movement of limb, which has a critical and vital role in reshaping the pathophysiology of lower extremity.
2. The baseline pigmentation of the leg (i.e., pre-treatment) should not be expected to reverse, especially within couple of years of treatment. The pigmentation, which presumably results from hemosiderin deposits that has been ongoing for several years, may not reverse at all. In best scenarios, it may reverse partially. It needs to be emphasized that reversing this pigmentation is not the goal of management. The prime objective is to reduce the impact of altered venous hemodynamics on the diseased limb and provide symptomatic relief.
3. The use of an 18-gauge venous access needle leaves a virtually undetectable scar on skin rendering this a minimal invasive procedure in a real sense.

COMPLICATIONS

Laser burns and DVT are the two most fear provoking complications of this procedure. But with the appropriate ultrasound guidance throughout the procedure, and perivenous tumescent anesthesia, both of which are negligible. There has been no report of cutaneous burns from laser ablation in recent past, and incidence of reported DVT is also minimal.

On the other hand, paresthesia can be encountered in practice. While saphenous paresthesia following GSV stripping is commonly seen[9], it is uncommon following laser ablation.[10] Similarly injury to sural nerve and tibial nerve have been reported following SSV stripping[11,12]. Proebstle et al reported paresthesia in 11% of patients that lasted 3-8 weeks, and none of them had significant concern.[13]

Sensation loss in the skin area innervated by the Saphenous nerve (SN) may be seen, which can be temporary or permanent, dependent on the extent of nerve damage[18,19].

In our practice, paresthesia was very rare, but when they do occur, are transient. Besides the thermal injury from laser, direct injury from injections of tumescent anesthesia can also cause nerve damage.

CONCEPT OF ENDOTHERMAL HEAT-INDUCED THROMBOSIS (EHIT)

With advent of endovenous ablation techniques, there were new set of conditions seen, and Endothermal heat-induced thrombosis (EHIT) was one of them. EHIT is different from of DVT, since the latter is a complication and not an expected outcome. EHIT is expected to happen due to inherent mechanism of action of endovenous ablation techniques, but should have its distribution in superficial venous system. But when it extends into deep system that may need attention. The extension into deep system can happened through gateway of SFJ, SPJ or perforators. So, in a way EHIT is a potential cause for DVT.

Mozes et al, in 2005, reported 7.7% of their cases had thrombus extending from GSV into CFV. In their cases though they started the GSV ablation 1 cm distal (i.e., peripheral) to the confluence of inferior epigastric vein and GSV. Their recommendation was to perform a 1-week follow up ultrasound to detect asymptomatic adverse events.[1]

One year earlier, in 2004, concern for DVT following RF Ablation was reported as a word of caution by Hingorani et al[2]. However, Min et al did not encounter this problem in 2003, in a largest report series of 499 patients at that time[3].

"Endovenous heat induced thrombus (EHIT) at the superficial-deep venous junction: a new post-treatment clinical entity, classification and patient treatment strategies" was presented at 18th Annual meeting of American Venous Forum in Feb 23, 2006 at Miami, Florida by Kabnick et al.[4] They classified EHIT into 4 class:

Class 1: venous thrombus extending up to superficial-deep vein junction (i.e. SFJ or SPJ). No extension into deep veins.

Class 2: venous thrombus extending into deep vein, but the thrombus is non-occlusive, and has a cross sectional diameter < 50 % of the venous lumen.

Class 3: venous thrombus extending into deep vein, but the thrombus is non-occlusive, and has a cross sectional diameter > 50 % of the venous lumen.

Class 4: Total occlusion of deep vein.

EHIT per se as a terminology is not listed in the multisociety consensus quality improvement guidelines 2007. In fact, they referred to this as "junction thrombus", and reported that the rate of this is widely variable. Interestingly, proximal extension of thrombus across SFJ is seen in 1% of cases if duplex US is performed in < 72 hours of ablation. The reported rates decrease if duplex US is performed later than 72 hours of ablation. This article mentions that it possible that this proximal extension of thrombus may be a self-limiting event without clinical implications. Data pooled from several sources reveal 0.3 % of incidence following laser ablation and 0.4% following RF ablation.[6] The incidence following SSV ablation is low and depends on SPJ anatomy.[7]

Lawrence et al came up with classification of proximal endovenous closure levels and treatment algorithm in 2010. They classified the closure levels 1 to 6, level 1 representing thrombus below the level of epigastric vein, and level 6 representing closure with thrombus extending into CFV, consistent with DVT. In their experience, patients with no history of DVT and GSV diameter < 8mm may not require a 48-72 hour follow up ultrasound, however, patients with history of DVT and GSV diameter > 8mm should undergo post procedure duplex exam.[8]

Sadek et al classified EHIT into 4 classes, class I being thrombus flush with SFJ, whereas class IV being a frank DVT[15].

The bottom-line is to understand the need for starting anticoagulant particularly in frank DVT and conditions when thrombus extension into CFV occupies majority of lumen. The non-occlusive thrombus eventually retracts in approximately 14 days, but a Low molecular weight heparin may have to be initiated[17].

EHIT associated DVT is relatively more frequent than non EHIT associated DVT[16,17].

In other words, you will find variable incidences of DVT mentioned in literature, that depends on two crucial factors:
- How is DVT defined (versus a Junctional thrombus or EHIT)
- When was the US performed following the procedure

Of note though, the EHIT regresses and virtually no post thrombotic syndrome or pulmonary embolism developing from EHIT have been noted. There has been debate on whether these thrombi need to be treated. Where there is a consensus, there is disagreement as well, in management of EHIT. Overall, EHIT 1 and EHIT 2 do not require anticoagulation. EHIT 3 may be observed, follow up and/or treated with anticoagulation. EHIT 4 may warrant treatment, although there may be some groups who disagree with that too.

REFERENCES:

1. Geza Mozes, Manju Kalra, Michele Carmo, Lori Swenson, Peter Gloviczki, Extension of saphenous thrombus into the femoral vein: A potential complication of new endovenous ablation techniques, Journal of Vascular Surgery, Volume 41, Issue 1, January 2005, Pages 130-135
2. Hingorani AP, Ascher E, Markevich N, Schutzer RW, Kallakuri S, Hou A, et al. Deep venous thrombosis after radiofrequency ablation of greater saphenous vein: a word of caution. J Vasc Surg 2004;40:500-4.
3. Min RJ, Khilnani N, Zimmet SE. Endovenous laser treatment of saphenous vein reflux: long-term results. J Vasc Interv Radiol 2003;14: 991-6.
4. Kabnick LS, Ombrellino M, Agis H, et al. Endovenous heat induced thrombus (EHIT) at the superficial-deep venous junction: a new post-treatment clinical entity, classification and patient treatment strategies [abstract]. Presented at the American Venous Forum 18th Annual Meeting; February 23, 2006; Miami, FL
5. Khilnani et al. Multi-society Consensus Quality Improvement Guidelines for the Treatment of Lowerextremity Superficial Venous Insufficiency with Endovenous Thermal Ablation from the Society of Interventional Radiology, Cardiovascular Interventional Radiological Society of Europe, American College of Phlebology, and Canadian Interventional Radiology Association. J Vasc Interv Radiol 2010; 21:14–31

6. Merchant RF, Kistner RL, Kabnick LS.Re: "Is there an increased risk for DVT after the Closure procedure? J Vasc Surg 2003; 38:628.
7. Gibson KD, Ferris BL, Polissar N,Neradilek B, Pepper D. Endovenous laser treatment of the short saphenous vein: efficacy and complications. J Vasc Surg 2007; 45:795–801.
8. Lawrence, Peter F. et al. Classification of proximal endovenous closure levels and treatment algorithm. J Vasc Surg 2010;52:388-93
9. Morrison C, Dalsing MC. Signs and symptoms of saphenous nerve injury after greater saphenous vein stripping: prevalence, severity and relevance for modern practice. J Vasc Surg 2003;38:886-90.
10. Kim HS, Nwankwo IJ, Hong K, McElgunn PSJ. Lower energy endovenous laser ablation of the great saphenous vein with 980 nm diode laser in continuous mode. Cardiovasc Intervent Radiol 2006;29:64-9.
11. Simonetti S, Bianchi S, Martinoli C. Neurophysiological and ultrasound findings in sural nerve lesions following stripping of the small saphenous vein. Muscle Nerve 1999;22:1724-6.
12. Kim HS, Nwankwo IJ, Hong K, McElgunn PSJ. Lower energy endovenous laser ablation of the great saphenous vein with 980 nm diode laser in ontinuous mode. Cardiovasc Intervent Radiol 2006; 29:64-9.
13. Proebstle TM, Gul D, Kargl A, Knop J. Endovenous Laser treatment of the lesser saphenous vein with a 940-nm diode laser: early results. Dermatol Surg 2003;29:357-61.
14. Ravi R, Rodriguez-Lopez JA, Traylor EA, Barrett DA, Ramaiah V, Diethrich EB. Endovenous ablation of incompetent saphenous veins: a large single-center experience. J Endovasc Ther 2006;13:244-8.
15. Sadek, Mikel et al. Increasing ablation distance peripheral to the saphenofemoral junction may result in a diminished rate of endothermal heat-induced thrombosis. Journal of Vascular Surgery: Venous and Lymphatic Disorders , Volume 1 , Issue 3 , 257 - 262

16. Meghan Dermody, Thomas F. O'Donnell, Ethan M. Balk, Complications of endovenous ablation in randomized controlled trials, Journal of Vascular Surgery: Venous and Lymphatic Disorders, Volume 1, Issue 4, October 2013, Pages 427-436.e1
17. Kane, K et al. The Incidence and Outcome of Endothermal Heat-induced Thrombosis after Endovenous Laser Ablation. Ann Vasc Surg. 2014 Oct;28(7):1744-50
18. L Veverkova´, VJedlic˘ka, PVlc˘ek andJKalac.The anatomical relationship between the saphenous nerve and the great saphenous vein. Phlebology 2011;26:114–118
19. Ramasastry SS, Dick GO, Futrell JW. Anatomy of the saphenous nerve: relevance to saphenous vein stripping. Am Surg. 1987 May;53(5):274-7.
20. Puggioni A, Kalra M, Carmo M, Mozes G, Gloviczki P. Endovenous laser therapy and radiofrequency ablation of the great saphenous vein: analysis of early efficacy and complications. J Vasc Surg 2005;42:488- 93.

Chapter 13

RECURRENCE OF VARICOSE VEINS

Varicose veins, due to its complex anatomy, variable pathophysiology and chronic nature, are a therapeutic challenge to any treating physician. Recurrence of varicosities and CVI invariably effects patient satisfaction and compliance, cost effectiveness and clinic workload. The ideal way of managing it is dealing with at the first instance. The ideal models serve as a lighthouse like guide but may not be practical in all cases.

The data from earlier studies has shown the effectiveness of dealing with it all at the first and same time has favorable outcome[1-5]. In a large series of patients who had concomitant treatment with endovenous laser and foam sclerotherapy at the same initial treatment session, there was 98% GSV success. 7% had incompetent perforators during the 1st year (majority within 3 months) and 3% during the next 2 years, i.e., 10% within first 3 years of combined treatment. Thereafter, over a period of additional 2 years, there were no new recurrences, and those 5% who presented with recurrence were amongst the same group of patients who had presented within first 3 years of treatment. The take home messages we have from these publications are:

- Deal with all the pathologic refluxes at the initial treatment session.
- Intense follow up ultrasound and clinic visits within first 3 months of treatment, and where indicated treat the recurrence at the earliest.
- Beyond 1 year, follow up annually or bi-annually for up to 3 years of treatment.
- Follow up after 3 years of treatment may not be required unless new symptoms develop.
- For those who had recurrence early on in 3 months, and within 3 years of treatment, are at increased risk of recurrence, and may need continued follow up.

Patterns of reflux responsible for recurrence

Perforator incompetence: The rate of perforator incompetence is higher in recurrent legs compared to those who present initially for treatment. These perforators could be anywhere, commonly seen in gaitor region of leg. However, incidence of thigh perforators is also high in recurrent limbs[7].

Deep venous insufficiency: It is more common in ulcerated legs.

GSV (groin) recurrence: This can be classified as[6]

- Types 1a – main stem recurrence. This is more of a concern in surgical approach, but could be seen in endovenous treatment due to unforeseen reasons. A representative example of such condition could be failure of laser fiber to emit energy due to technical reasons.
- Type 1b- tributary filling up GSV. If a tributary refluxed into stump of central aspect of GSV (which is closer to SFJ) that has been left out intentionally (as you may recall from the procedure chapter),

which then happens to communicate with other superficial vein of lower extremity, could potentially result recurrence of varicosities.
- Type 1c- Neovascularisation or formation of new vascular channels[8,9,10]. The majority of recurrences are secondary to neovascularization.

SPJ incompetence: more common in ulcerated legs.

NOTE: Multiple sites of incompetence are more commonly seen in recurrences as opposed to one single site.

Management of recurrence
1. Identify the anatomical site of recurrence on ultrasound.
2. Evaluate and assess patient's compliance with compression stockings, calf exercises and body weight optimization.
3. Foam sclerotherapy has been our choice to deal with these recurrences, which is minimally invasive.
4.

REFERENCES:

1. M.I. Bhalla, N. Bhalla. Treatment of lower limb varicosities with combined use of endovenous laser and sclerosant at the same instance - A unique study of 286 patients. Journal of Vascular and Interventional Radiology, Feb 2010; 21(2): S70
2. M. Bhalla, N. Bhalla. Concomitant use of endovenous laser and foamed sclerosant for treatment of lower limb varicosities. Insights Imaging, 2011; 2(1): S275
3. M.I. Bhalla, N. Bhalla. Concomitant use of endovenous laser and foamed sclerosant in the treatment of lower limb varicosities: 3 year follow-up results. Journal of Vascular and Interventional Radiology, 2011; 22(3): S18–S19

4. M.I. Bhalla, N. Bhalla. Concomitant use of endovenous laser and foamed sclerosant in treatment of lower limb varicosities: 5 year follow-up results. Journal of Vascular and Interventional Radiology, March 2012; 23(3): S115
5. M. Bhalla, N. Bhalla, H. Vasavada Concomitant use of endovenous laser and foamed sclerosant in treatment of lower limb varicosities: 3 year follow-up results. Insights Imaging, 2012; 3(1): S230
6. Stonebridge PA, Chalmers N, Beggs I, Bradbury AW, Ruckley CV. Recurrent varicose veins: a varicographic analysis leading to a new practical classification. Br J Surg 1995; 82: 60±62.
7. Wong JK[1], Duncan JL, Nichols DM. Whole-leg duplex mapping for varicose veins: observations on patterns of reflux in recurrent and primary legs, with clinical correlation. Eur J Vasc Endovasc Surg. 2003 Mar;25(3):267-75.
8. Glass GM. Neovascularization in recurrence of varices of the great saphenous vein in the groin: phlebography. Angiology 1988;39:577-82.
9. Jones L, Braithwaite BD, Selwyn D, Cooke S, Earnshaw JJ. Neovascularisation is the principal cause of varicose vein recurrence: results of a randomised trial of stripping the long saphenous vein. Eur J Vasc Endovasc Surg 1996;12:442-5.
10. Nyamekye I, Shephard NA, Davies B, Heather BP, Earnshaw JJ. Clinicopathological evidence that neovascularisation is a cause of recurrent varicose veins. Eur J Vasc Endovasc Surg 1998;15:412-5.

Conclusion

Endovenous laser ablation of varicose veins is:

- ✓ Safe
- ✓ Effective
- ✓ Durable results
- ✓ Can be performed concomitantly
- ✓ Can be performed as outpatient
- ✓ Acceptable low incidence of nerve injury
- ✓ Acceptable low incidence of DVT

EVLT is a reliable and efficient new technique to treat varicose veins. Even a concomitant open ulcer is no contraindication for using EVLT However, precautions such as coverage with film dressings or, even better, total exclusion of such open wounds from the operating field by the use of surgical drapes, should be taken to minimize the risk of infection. In addition, perioperative antibiotics, possibly based on ulcer culture results, should likely be strongly considered. Finally, it is crucial that the physician who performs this type of treatment should be able to master every possible complication and should not hesitate to perform even aggressive surgical intervention.

Significant improvements in physician-measured outcomes such as venous clinical severity scores (VCSS) scores and air-plethysmography (APG) have been reported following endovenous ablation technique.

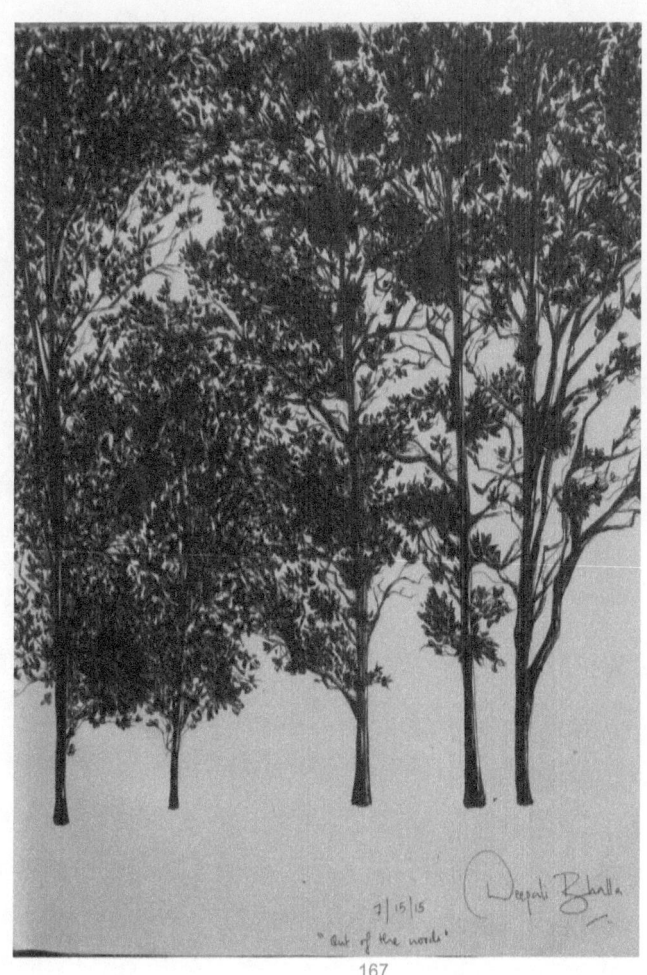

www.ingramcontent.com/pod-product-compliance
Lightning Source LLC
Chambersburg PA
CBHW031631210526
45464CB00004B/1854